CONTENTS

SUSAN V. GARSTANG, MD, Assistant Professor, Department of Physical Medicine and Rehabilitation, University of Medicine and Dentistry of New Jersey, New Jersey Medical School, Newark, New Jersey

DAVID R. GATER, Jr, MD, PhD, Chief, Spinal Cord Injury and Disorders Center, Hunter Holmes McGuire Veterans Affairs Medical Center; Professor, Department of Physical Medicine and Rehabilitation, Virginia Commonwealth University, Richmond, Virginia

SUSAN J. HARKEMA, PhD, Associate Professor and Owsley B. Frazier Chair of Neurological Rehabilitation, Department of Neurological Surgery, Kentucky Spinal Cord Injury Research Center, University of Louisville and Frazier Rehab Institute, Louisville, Kentucky

CHESTER H. HO, MD, Chief, Spinal Cord Injury, Principal Investigator, Cleveland Functional Electrical Stimulation Center, Principal Investigator, Advanced Platform Technology Center, Louis Stokes Cleveland Department of Veterans Affairs Medical Center; and Senior Research Associate, Department of Orthopaedics, Case Western Reserve University, Cleveland, Ohio

SHERRI L. LAVELA, MPH, MBA, Research Scientist, Center for Management of Complex Chronic Care; Research Investigator, Spinal Cord Injury Quality Enhancement Research Initiative, Department of Veterans Affairs, Edward Hines Jr. Veterans Affairs Hospital, Hines, Illinois; Gerontological Research Fellow, United States National Institutes of Health, National Institute on Aging; and Center for Research on Health and Aging, Institute for Health Research and Policy, Chicago, Illinois

TIMOTHY D. LAVIS, MD, Carolinas Rehabilitation, Carolinas Medical Center, Charlotte, North Carolina

STACEY A. MILLER-SMITH, MD, Resident, Department of Physical Medicine and Rehabilitation, University of Medicine and Dentistry of New Jersey, New Jersey Medical School, Newark, New Jersey

GREGORY SAMSON, MD, Spinal Cord Injury Fellow, Department of Rehabilitation Medicine, Leonard M. Miller School of Medicine, Miami, Florida

WILLIAM M. SCELZA, MD, Carolinas Rehabilitation, Carolinas Medical Center, Charlotte, North Carolina

PHILIP M. ULLRICH, PhD, Veterans Affairs Puget Sound Healthcare System, Seattle, Washington

FRANCES M. WEAVER, PhD, Deputy Director, Center for Management of Complex Chronic Care; Research Director, Spinal Cord Injury Quality Enhancement Research Initiative, Department of Veterans Affairs, Edward Hines Jr. Veterans Affairs Hospital, Hines, Illinois; and Research Associate Professor, Neurology Department, Northwestern University, Chicago, Illinois

CONSULTING EDITOR

GEORGE H. KRAFT, MD, MS, Alvord Professor of Multiple Sclerosis Research, Professor, Rehabilitation Medicine, Adjunct Professor, Neurology, University of Washington, Seattle, Washington

GUEST EDITORS

BARRY GOLDSTEIN, MD, PhD, Associate Chief Consultant, Spinal Cord Injury and Disorders Services, Department of Veterans Affairs; Professor, Department of Rehabilitation Medicine, University of Washington, Seattle, Washington

MARGARET C. HAMMOND, MD, Associate Chief Consultant, Spinal Cord Injury and Disorders Services, Department of Veterans Affairs; Professor, Department of Rehabilitation Medicine, University of Washington, Seattle, Washington

CONTRIBUTORS

ANDREA L. BEHRMAN, PhD, Associate Professor, Department of Physical Therapy, College of Public Health and Health Professions, University of Florida; and Research Health Scientist, Veterans Affairs Brain Rehabilitation Research Center, Malcom Randall Veterans Affairs Medical Center, Gainesville, Florida

WILLIAM L. BOCKENEK, MD, Medical Director, Carolinas Rehabilitation; Chairman, Department of Physical Medicine and Rehabilitation, Carolinas Medical Center, Charlotte, North Carolina

KATH BOGIE, DPhil, Principal Investigator, Cleveland Functional Electrical Stimulation Center; Principal Investigator, Advanced Platform Technology Center, Louis Stokes Cleveland Department of Veterans Affairs Medical Center; and Senior Research Associate, Department of Orthopaedics, Case Western Reserve University, Cleveland, Ohio

STEPHEN P. BURNS, MD, Staff Physician, Spinal Cord Injury Service, Veterans Affairs Puget Sound Health Care System; Associate Professor, Department of Rehabilitation Medicine, University of Washington; Section Head for Rehabilitation, Harborview Injury Prevention and Research Center, Seattle, Washington

DIANA D. CARDENAS, MD, MHA, Professor and Chair, Department of Rehabilitation Medicine, Leonard M. Miller School of Medicine, Miami, Florida; and Lois Pope LIFE Center, Miami, Florida

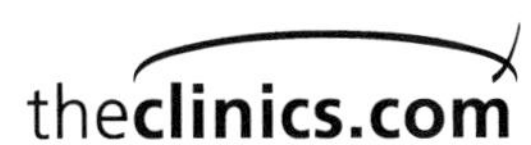

PHYSICAL MEDICINE AND REHABILITATION CLINICS OF NORTH AMERICA

Topics in Spinal Cord Injury Medicine

GUEST EDITORS
Barry Goldstein, MD, PhD
Margaret C. Hammond, MD

CONSULTING EDITOR
George H. Kraft, MD, MS

May 2007 • Volume 18 • Number 2

SAUNDERS

An Imprint of Elsevier, Inc.
PHILADELPHIA LONDON TORONTO MONTREAL SYDNEY TOKYO

W.B. SAUNDERS COMPANY
A Division of Elsevier Inc.

1600 John F. Kennedy Blvd. • Suite 1800 • Philadelphia, Pennsylvania 19103

http://www.theclinics.com

PHYSICAL MEDICINE AND REHABILITATION CLINICS OF NORTH AMERICA
May 2007
Editor: Debora Dellapena

Volume 18, Number 2
ISSN 1047-9651
ISBN 1-4160-4746-8
978-1-4160-4746-9

Physical Medicine and Rehabilitation Clinics of North America (ISSN 1047-9651) is published quarterly by Elsevier Inc., 360 Park Avenue South, New York, NY 10010-1710. Months of publication are February, May, August, and November. Business and Editorial Offices: 1600 John F. Kennedy Blvd., Suite 1800, Philadelphia, PA 19103-2899. Customer Service Office: 6277 Sea Harbor Drive, Orlando, FL 32887-4800. Periodicals postage paid at New York, NY and additional mailing offices. Subscription price per year is $179.00 (US individuals), $275.00 (US institutions), $90.00 (US students), $218.00 (Canadian individuals), $352.00 (Canadian institutions), $123.00 (Canadian students), $252.00 (foreign individuals), $352.00 (foreign institutions), and $123.00 (foreign students). Foreign air speed delivery is included in all *Clinics* subscription prices. All prices are subject to change without notice. POSTMASTER: Send address changes to *Physical Medicine and Rehabilitation Clinics of North America*, Elsevier Periodicals Customer Service, 6277 Sea Harbor Drive, Orlando, FL 32887-4800. **Customer Service: 1-800-654-2452 (US). From outside of the US, call 1-407-345-4000.**

Physical Medicine and Rehabilitation Clinics of North America is indexed in *Excerpta Medica, Index Medicus, Cinahl*, and *Cumulative Index to Nursing and Allied Health Literature.*

Printed in the United States of America.

FORTHCOMING ISSUES

August 2007

Gender Specific Medicine:
The Physiatrist and Women's Health
Sheila A. Dugan, MD and
Heidi Prather, DO, *Guest Editors*

November 2007

Up-to-Date Advances in Rehabilitation
Seema Khurana, DO, *Guest Editor*

February 2008

Neuromuscular Complications
of Systemic Conditions
Kathryn Stolp, MD, *Guest Editor*

May 2008

Child and Adolescent Sports Injuries
Brain Krabak, MD, MBA, *Guest Editor*

RECENT ISSUES

February 2007

Traumatic Brain Injury: New Directions
and Treatment Approaches
James A. Young, MD, *Guest Editor*

November 2006

Performing Arts Medicine
Seneca A. Storm, MD, *Guest Editor*

August 2006

Sports Medicine
Gregory A. Strock, MD and
Ralph Buschbacher, MD, *Guest Editors*

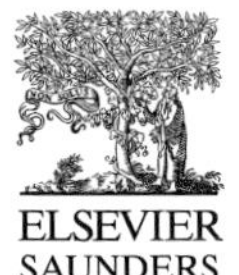
ELSEVIER
SAUNDERS

Phys Med Rehabil Clin N Am
18 (2007) ix–x

PHYSICAL MEDICINE
AND REHABILITATION
CLINICS OF
NORTH AMERICA

Foreword

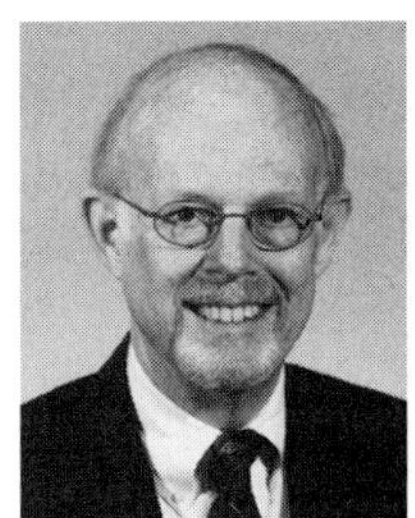

George H. Kraft, MD, MS
Consulting Editor

It has been some time since we had an issue on spinal cord injury (SCI). Because of shifting interests in the field of physical medicine and rehabilitation—and an increased focus on musculoskeletal/sports medicine—we have recently been focusing more on that area. However, SCI still retains an important place in our field (it is, indeed, a subspecialty of the American Board of Physical Medicine and Rehabilitation), and it is time that the *Physical Medicine and Rehabilitation Clinics of North America* devotes another issue to SCI medicine.

This may be the place for a little historical perspective: During World War II, Dr. Howard Rusk—the father of rehabilitation, but an internist by training—assumed the position as the person responsible for the care of severely injured servicemen. He had no model for this care, but instinctively knew that they should not be left to spend the remainder of their lives in a custodial institution. Many were amputees, but many were also SCI patients.

At that time, patients with SCI were kept in bed in nursing homes, quickly developed skin breakdown and subsequent septicemia, or developed and died of urinary tract infections. Their postinjury life was predictably short. Because the internal organ system often affected was the kidneys, urologists often managed their care. Dr. Rusk thought there must be a better way to care for these servicemen, and rehabilitation medicine was created.

So the problems of management of SCI even preceded the development of the field of physical medicine and rehabilitation. Traditionally, military

1047-9651/07/$ - see front matter
doi:10.1016/j.pmr.2007.03.006

action has been a stimulus for the development of SCI care. In fact, the Paralyzed Veterans of America (PVA) has been at the forefront of developing care systems for injured servicemen. Their focus has been not only during their period in the military but also in the postmilitary period. Through the many efforts of the PVA, as well as others, the SCI program in the Veterans Affairs was established.

It should be no surprise, then, that many of the pre-eminent SCI programs are in the Veterans Affairs system. That is why I am so pleased that Dr. Margaret Hammond, Professor and Chief Consultant on SCI, and her colleague, Dr. Barry Goldstein, Professor of Rehabilitation Medicine and Associate Chief Consultant, agreed to act as Guest Editors for this issue. Through their intimate understanding of the SCI field and its resources, they have collected articles on important management issues of SCI care.

I am convinced that this brief issue will provide an important update for physicians managing SCI patients. Thank you to Dr. Hammond and Dr. Goldstein for organizing it.

George H. Kraft, MD, MS
University of Washington
School of Medicine
1959 NE Pacific St., Box 356490
Seattle, WA 98195-6490, USA

E-mail address: ghkraft@u.washington.edu

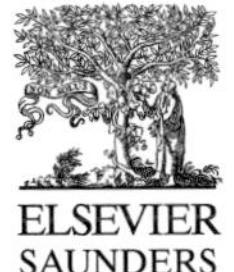
ELSEVIER
SAUNDERS

Phys Med Rehabil Clin N Am
18 (2007) xi–xii

PHYSICAL MEDICINE
AND REHABILITATION
CLINICS OF
NORTH AMERICA

Preface

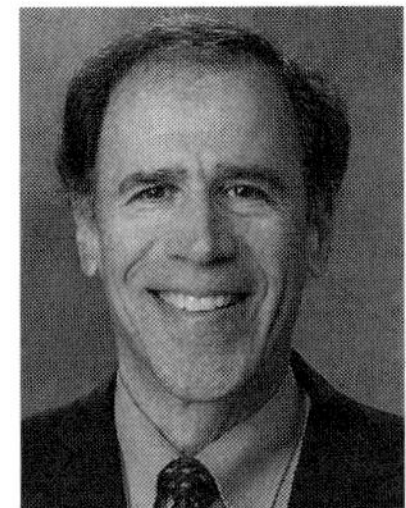

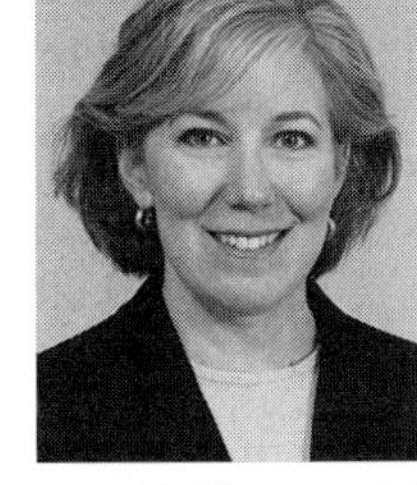

Barry Goldstein, MD, PhD Margaret C. Hammond, MD
Guest Editors

It has been 7 years since the *Physical Medicine and Rehabilitation Clinics of North America* have devoted an issue to spinal cord medicine. Many changes have taken place since then in the overall understanding of neuroplasticity and other basic mechanisms of recovery, technologic advances to improve function, equipment, and access, a better appreciation of comorbid problems following spinal cord injury (SCI), and preventive care services. There has been continued progress in developing an evidence base in spinal cord medicine, and there have been several new clinical practice guidelines published by the Consortium for Spinal Cord Medicine.

In this issue, several of the more vexing problems in spinal cord medicine are discussed. Behrman and Harkema review the recent literature on activity-based therapies that target recovery of standing and walking based on physical rehabilitation interventions to facilitate recovery. Several articles focus on new developments in the diagnosis and treatment of complex comorbid conditions. Ho and Bogie bring a new focus to the area of pressure ulcer prevention and treatment by concentrating on conceptual approaches, technologic advances, and methodologies that are on the horizon for this frustrating problem. Burns reviews management principles for prevention and treatment of respiratory infections in persons with SCI, an important area because respiratory disorders remain the leading cause of death during the acute and chronic periods after SCI. Ullrich discusses chronic pain and reviews what is known and gaps in

The work by the *Guest Editors* represents views of the editors (Goldstein and Hammond), and does not necessarily reflect the opinions of the Department of Veterans Affairs.

1047-9651/07/$ - see front matter © 2007 Published by Elsevier Inc.
doi:10.1016/j.pmr.2007.04.001

our knowledge in this complex area. Several articles reflect an increasing awareness of comorbid problems related to metabolic disorders and the increased lifespan of people who live with SCI. Lavis and colleagues discuss cardiovascular health and fitness, Gater evaluates obesity, and Weaver and LaVela discuss the importance of prevention and health maintenance when living with chronic conditions that follow SCI. Impairments in autonomic function remain a complex issue after SCI. Garstang and Miller-Smith discuss the manifestations of autonomic dysfunction, while Samson and Cardenas review management of the neurogenic bladder.

By taking on some of the more complex problems that follow an SCI, we hope that this issue provides both a review of current knowledge and stimulates new ideas. We wish to thank the authors for the time, energy, and passion that they put into this effort. Their commitment in caring for people with a SCI is inspirational. We also wish to recognize the pioneers in SCI, to whom we are indebted for their vision and insight. We truly stand on their shoulders.

Barry Goldstein, MD, PhD
Margaret C. Hammond, MD
Spinal Cord Injury and Disorders Services (128 NAT)
Department of Veterans Affairs
1660 S. Columbian Way, Seattle, WA 98108-1597, USA
Department of Rehabilitation Medicine, University of Washington
Seattle, WA, USA

E-mail address: barry.goldstein@va.gov

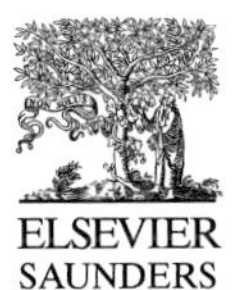

ELSEVIER
SAUNDERS

Phys Med Rehabil Clin N Am
18 (2007) 183–202

PHYSICAL MEDICINE
AND REHABILITATION
CLINICS OF
NORTH AMERICA

Physical Rehabilitation as an Agent for Recovery After Spinal Cord Injury

Andrea L. Behrman, PhD[a,b,*], Susan J. Harkema, PhD[c]

[a]*Department of Physical Therapy, College of Public Health and Health Professions, P.O. Box 100154, University of Florida, Gainesville, FL 32610-0154, USA*
[b]*VA Brain Rehabilitation Research Center (151A), Malcom Randall VA Medical Center, 1601 SW Archer Road, Gainesville, FL 32608, USA*
[c]*Department of Neurological Surgery, Kentucky Spinal Cord Injury Research Center, University of Louisville and Frazier Rehab Institute, 220 Abraham Flexner Way, Louisville, KY 40402, USA*

Clinicians, including physicians and therapists, have developed prognostications for expectations of functional outcomes after spinal cord injury (SCI) [1]. Outcomes expected 1 year after injury are based on the initial level of injury and the initial degree of voluntary strength of the muscles below the level of injury [2]. Rehabilitation planning and outcomes relative to independence, self-care, and mobility are based on the degree of neurologic impairment assessed by a standardized neurologic evaluation developed by the American Spinal Injury Association (ASIA) and termed the ASIA Impairment Scale (AIS) [1,3–6]. The magnitude and rate of recovery depends on the initial injury severity and whether it is complete (AIS A), sensory incomplete (AIS B), or motor incomplete (AIS C or D) [3,7–12], with motor incomplete injuries showing a more rapid rate of recovery. The rate of recovery is measured by the relative change in the motor and sensory scores over time and declines substantially after 6 months to 1 year after SCI [13].

Dr. Behrman acknowledges support from NIH (K-01 HD01348-01), VA RR and D grant F21821C, and the America Paraplegia Society for her research.

Dr. Harkema acknowledges support from the NeuroRecovery Network funded by the Christopher and Dana Reeve Foundation through Grant/Cooperative Agreement Number U10/CCU220379 between CDRF and Centers for Disease Control and Prevention (CDC). Its contents are solely the responsibility of the authors and do not necessarily represent the official views of the CDC. Her work is also funded by NIH grants: R01NS049209, P01NS16333.

* Corresponding author. Department of Physical Therapy, College of Public Health and Health Professions, P.O. Box 100154, University of Florida, Gainesville, FL 32610-0154.

E-mail address: abehrman@phhp.ufl.edu (A.L. Behrman).

doi:10.1016/j.pmr.2007.02.002

The loss of standing and walking after human SCI has been attributed to the dominance of supraspinal mechanisms over spinal mechanisms in the control of locomotion [14–17]. Thus, pharmacologic [18–22] and surgical interventions [23,24] have been the predominant focus for altering the course of natural recovery by improving functional outcomes after SCI. These interventions are associated with medical management during the acute phase after SCI to diminish the damaging sequelae of acute SCI including swelling or cord impingement. From this vantage point, recovery has been equated with improvements according to the AIS evaluation of voluntary strength and sensation and associated functional gains in abilities [25].

Physical rehabilitation as compensation for irremediable deficits and new skill development

Physical rehabilitation after SCI has relied substantially on compensatory strategies for identified nonremediable impairments and deficits, because significant recovery of motor function was not expected beyond that defined by the clinical assessments. In addition, health care provider limitations have significantly reduced the number and duration of therapy sessions necessitating that therapists target immediate patient needs in preparation for discharge [26]. New behavioral strategies are taught to accomplish tasks including rolling over in bed, getting up from the floor to a chair, and transferring in and out of a wheelchair [27–29]. Each of these new skills relies on strengthening of muscles above the level of the lesion and use leverage, momentum, and substitution to aid in moving a weak or paralyzed body for new mobility skills [27,30]. These individuals with SCI usually do not recover their preinjury ability to roll over in bed, dress, stand up, grasp a glass, or get in and out of a car, but instead develop an entirely new repertoire of movement strategies to accomplish daily activities or they remain dependent on others for assistance. The process of learning these new skills requires practice and repetition, and the ability to problem-solve to find unique approaches to maneuver successfully through the myriad of circumstances and environments of daily life.

Additionally, wheelchairs, assistive devices, and braces are incorporated into the new skill learning associated with mobility [27–29]. Wheelchairs offer a means of alternative mobility from a seated position and require the acquisition of new skills to propel and maneuver the equipment using the arms, head, chin, breath, or hand controls. Leg braces and assistive devices provide stability for joints that cannot be activated voluntarily and when muscle strength is not adequate to support upright posture during standing and walking. For example, walking using leg braces and a walker is highly dependent on voluntary motor control above the level of lesion and assistance from the devices to achieve a new approach to stability and mobility. However, accomplishing the activities of daily living using compensatory strategies is not equivalent to recovery of motor control that restores preinjury capabilities (ie, walking upright at normal speed, negotiating obstacles with balance responses, and climbing stairs) [31–38].

Conventional gait training post-SCI is routinely conducted over ground. A tilt table, parallel bars, assistive devices, and braces are all used to achieve upright standing and compensate for lower extremity and trunk weakness or paralysis and possibly upper extremity weakness [27–29]. Walking in the overground environment is certainly the end goal and thus readily experienced in this environment. However, without substantial evidence of recovery of voluntary control below the lesion, those with SCI are instructed to achieve walking via compensatory strategies. These strategies use passive external lower extremity support (braces) and upper extremity weight bearing (assistive devices) to overcome sensorimotor deficits.

Emerging physical rehabilitation: activity-based therapies for recovery of function after spinal chord injury

Evidence from basic and applied science for activity-dependent plasticity of the neural axis, including the spinal cord, has provided a new perspective on the role of physical rehabilitation for the recovery of motor function after SCI [39–43]. Research studies in animals and humans that have found that retraining after SCI using the intrinsic physiologic properties of the nervous system can facilitate the recovery of function [41,42,44,45]. This potential for retraining is based on activity-dependent plasticity driven by repetitive task-specific sensory input to spinal networks. These studies show that the spinal cord integrates supraspinal and afferent information and with repetitive practice can improve motor output. With the translation of these scientific findings to the human condition, rehabilitation strategies emerged that use the intrinsic processes of the nervous system in response to task-specific activity to advance and improve recovery of function after SCI [39,40,46–49].

Activity-based therapy has recently been promoted at prominent rehabilitation centers in the United States to describe their therapeutic interventions [50–57]. However, the term is used ubiquitously often to describe the usual compensatory approaches to regain the ability to perform specific functions. In the scientific literature, *activity-dependent plasticity* is a term that has general consensus to indicate changes in the nervous or muscular systems that are driven by repetitive activity [58]. Thus, activity-based therapy specifically refers to interventions that provide activation of the neuromuscular system below the level of lesion with the goal of retraining the nervous system to recover a specific motor task. The approach is to evaluate the neurophysiologic state below the level of lesion [59–62] and phase of recovery and then use repetitive practice of the desired task to functionally reorganize the nervous system [41]. So an activity-based therapy is an intervention that results in neuromuscular activation below the level of the lesion to promote recovery of motor function with the activation driven by the nervous system as most desirable.

The most prominent and well-developed activity-based therapy (physical rehabilitation) to date is "locomotor training" (LT) [39–41,46,47]. A series of guiding principles for training has emerged in the translation of findings from basic science to the human condition [39–41,46,47,63]. Scientists, examining the role of the spinal cord in controlling walking, discovered that cats with complete mid-thoracic transactions of the spinal cord could generate a stepping response after intense daily and long-term practice of the task of walking. Walking was facilitated by manual trainers assisting limb flexion, reflex extensor activity via pinching of the tail and/or anal region, while providing partial body weight support to the trunk by a sling suspension [64]. Training involved optimizing normative stepping parameters including speed of stepping and appropriate kinematics and kinetics.

Guiding principles of locomotor training

Guidelines for locomotor training provide a framework for clinical decision making, as well as a reference point for evaluating the potential application of any new modality, equipment, or therapeutic component within LT. Clinical choices can be made that are consistent with the framework (ie, no weight bearing on the upper extremities during training on the treadmill) for recovery or that are inconsistent (ie, use of a long-leg brace) and reflect a choice for compensation. Although training protocols used by researchers and clinicians vary [46], these guidelines represent a structured translation from basic science evidence for the neural control of walking to therapeutic principles for retraining walking. These guidelines will continue to be refined and clarified [65,66] as research advances the science of locomotor training.

Four guiding principles of LT [46,47] are built on the premise of robustly approximating the sensorimotor experience of walking [42] through repetitive practice:

1. Maximize load bearing by the lower extremities and minimize load bearing by the upper extremities. Increases in limb electromyographic amplitude are associated with increasing load bearing in both animals and humans after SCI as well as able-bodied individuals [67,68]. This physiologic response to the sensory input associated with load bearing and translated into a guiding principle provides the opportunity to improve activation in muscles that under voluntary conditions (ie, manual muscle testing) are weak or do not produce a contraction. Visintin and Barbeau [34] observed that shared load bearing between the upper and lower limbs diminished electromyographic (EMG) activity in the lower limbs. In contrast, providing partial body weight support through vertical suspension produced a relative increase in lower limb EMG activity. Thus, minimizing upper limb loading during retraining by use of hand rails or parallel bars is discouraged, and increasing vertical load bearing through the legs is encouraged.

2. Optimize the sensory cues for walking. Normal walking speed for an adult ranges from 0.8 to 1.2 m/s [69] and affords the spatial-temporal sequence of inputs that contribute to the characteristic sensorimotor experience of walking. Whether normal walking speed is a necessary component to the ensemble of activity-dependent experience producing a beneficial effect of LT continues to be a question of researchers [70]. Beres-Jones and Harkema [71] and Lunenburger and colleagues [72] observed velocity-dependent modulation of EMG activity in persons with both incomplete and complete SCI and able-bodied individuals. Again, in an effort to increase muscle activation, the higher speeds may provide a stronger stimulus response.
3. Optimize the kinematics (ie, trunk and extremities) for each motor task. One critical kinematic component to successful walking is the transition from stance to swing. This transition may be neurally activated by the sensory input associated with hip extension (relative to an upright trunk) and limb load bearing (muscle/tendon stretch, proprioception, cutaneous input), followed by unloading of the limb while transferring weight to the other limb. These two sensory elements, extension and load, are part of the essential ensemble of afferent input affording the transition and generation of activity from stance to swing or extension to flexion [73,74]. Incorporating these elements into the training regime is critical to initiating and generating flexion in the gait cycle.Because the arms typically swing in reciprocal coordination with the lower limbs while walking, this automatic pattern and kinematic component may be of benefit in achieving a more complete sensory experience of walking. Furthermore, armswing may contribute to activity-dependent plasticity [75] and development of appropriate balance responses and is thus encouraged by some researchers and trainers [46,47] as opposed to a supportive function by the upper extremities.
4. Maximize recovery strategies and minimize compensation strategies. Recovery strategies promote use of the inherent biology of the nervous system to generate motor responses within the usual kinematic framework. Visintin and Barbeau [34] concluded that using parallel bars for upper extremity (UE) support produced a forward flexed trunk, asymmetry in gait, and use of compensatory strategies for swing initiation such as "hip-hiking" (eg, the trunk flexes laterally while raising the hip and advancing the leg forward with the knee extended). By comparison, vertical support provided a more upright trunk, hip extension and loading promoting the transition from stance to swing, and relatively less compensatory movement strategies while walking. The latter experience would be more consistent with the LT principles and a more appropriate choice for retraining the nervous system. Throughout LT, individuals are encouraged to attempt movements but are assisted, as needed, to perform them to achieve the task-specific sensory experience, ie, thus, movement without compensatory pattern.

Locomotor training environments and progression

Body weight support and treadmill environment

For LT, the primary retraining for the capacity to walk occurs in the treadmill environment. Barbeau and colleagues [76] first extended the training environment of the animal model studies to clinical application for humans after SCI. He and his colleagues developed an overhead suspension system attached to a body harness worn by the subject while walking on a treadmill [76,77]. Early experiments assessed the simple effect of body weight support (BWS) on gait in able-bodied subjects [76,77]. Studies continue today to examine the effect of types of BWS and harness systems [78–80]. Manufacturers of BWS systems offer varying specifications of control that offer relatively different approximations of the body's center of mass during walking and the ground reaction forces during loading and propulsion [81].

The body weight support and treadmill (BWST) environment provides a permissive environment in that it may afford the individual a walking experience that more closely approximates the actual sensorimotor pattern of walking when compared with walking overground. In addition, the BWST environment provides a heightened degree of control and quantification of the sensorimotor experience relative to treadmill speed and BWS. In this environment, the spinal and supraspinal networks for locomotion are functionally reorganized. This new training environment meets the demands of retraining by affording the sensory experience of walking as well as the necessary intensity of repetition and practice [41]. The number of steps that may be achieved in one session in this environment when compared with overground may be a critical component to successful retraining of the nervous system. In some instances, BWS may not be necessary and simply the treadmill may provide an adequate stimulus to practice walking while approximating normal walking speeds [47].

Many individuals, however, cannot move a limb or do so awkwardly with considerable physical and cognitive effort to achieve a step and often a kinematic incorrect step. These individuals require manual assistance of trainers to (1) provide upright trunk support, (2) facilitate flexion and extension patterns of limb activity, and (3) promote pelvic rotation and weight transfer during loading of the stance limb [46,47,63,82]. Trainers in the clinical context provide assistance as needed to promote activation of muscles within the context of the limb trajectories for the stepping pattern, pelvic movement, and trunk control. Proper ergonomic seats for the trainers at the level of the treadmill with back and leg supports are a necessity for the repetitive task of manual training [81]. A more detailed explanation of manual assistance is provided in several case study reports [46,47].

Robotic-assistance was designed to provide an automated system of moving the legs in a stepping pattern on a treadmill using BWS [83–86]. A robot consisting of an exoskeleton with motors at the hip and knee joints and integrated with the BWST provides a consistent pattern of flexion and extension for stepping. Pelvic and trunk stabilization are provided via straps and supports that minimize or eliminate movement. As a computer-controlled system, BWS and treadmill speed can be varied in conjunction with the spatial-temporal pattern controlled by hip and knee range of motion (ROM) and step length. The robotic system may offer greater consistency of limb trajectories for patterned stepping by eliminating therapist fatigue and thus provides a greater duration of therapy. However, the robotic assistance may provide a more stereotyped and consistent pattern of limb movement than the alternative, manual assistance. In addition, manual assistance allows for real-time decision-making by the therapist to adapt immediately to the patient to achieve proper limb kinematics and the spatio-temporal pattern. Further studies are needed to identify the most efficacious approach to providing the needed assistance during retraining and the potential differential effects in the process of recovery of function.

LT-overground

With the ultimate aim of LT to improve or restore walking ability overground, skills acquired in the treadmill environment must be assessed and translated to overground. The same guiding principles are extended from the treadmill to overground environment. Thus, use of the LT principles has ramifications for how training occurs in the treadmill and overground environments, both in the clinic and at home. For instance, to maintain hip extension while walking with an assistive device introduced overground, the individual must maintain an upright posture and minimize the upper extremity load-bearing on a device. Translation of the training principles beyond the treadmill environment has been developed and studied as an integral component of a locomotor training program by several researchers [47,87–89].

Furthermore, a new generation of assistive devices and options for use of standard devices may develop that are consistent with the goal of recovery of function. For instance, use of a walking or trekking pole (or pair) may promote a more upright posture with minimal balance and weight-bearing support in contrast to the conventional use of a single point cane. The standard four-point walker used for gait training when reversed (with the cross bar positioned behind the patient and open-end forward of the patient) may also promote an upright posture with less weight bearing on the arms.

LT as a rehabilitative strategy has been successful for many people with acute and chronic incomplete SCI; however, varied results are reported [46,63,66,85,89–95]. This variability may be caused by the differences among therapists in the relative level of knowledge of the principles underlying retraining of the nervous system, their skill in applying these principles, and the effectiveness of the decisions that are made to progress the recovery as well as the intensity and duration of the intervention. Therapists who are aware of the potential of the spinal networks and sensory signals to modulate muscle activation patterns will have the best chance of optimizing LT for their patients. Implementing LT in the clinic is in the relatively early stages of development, and future efforts should focus on education, training, and establishing standards. Optimizing the protocols for specific patient populations is continually evolving as we simultaneously learn more from ongoing studies. Efficient and effective translation of scientific and clinical evidence to routine clinical practice will take collaborative efforts among scientists, clinicians, and administrators.

Electrical stimulation to activate the neuromuscular system during walking and standing

Although LT induces neuromuscular activation below the lesion by providing the appropriate sensory information back to the nervous system, use of electrical stimulation achieves standing and walking by stimulating muscles that are impaired. Electrical stimulation to the common peroneal nerve to generate a flexor withdrawal response is often used during walking on the treadmill with BWS and overground. The stimulation and flexor response are timed to synchronize with the initiation of the swing phase. Training with swing phase assist using electrical stimulation while walking in the BWST environment has improved walking speed in individuals with AIS C classification and asymmetrical LE function [66,91]. Similarly, Fung and Barbeau [96] used repeated conditioning of the H-reflex to generate a similar flexor response coordinated with the transition from terminal stance to swing in individuals with incomplete SCI. Electrical stimulation is an alternative means of activating sensory afferents and generating flexor responses within the task of walking. Removal of the electrical stimulation has resulted in sustained improvements and thus represents relatively permanent adaptability by the nervous system in individuals who could already take steps [66,91]. In addition to use of electrical stimulation to generate a flexor response, electrical stimulation has been also used to assist knee extension during the stance phase of walking [97,98]. Functional electrical stimulation (FES) has an immediate effect on the gait and serves as a neuroprosthesis. Long-term use of FES-assisted walking has also resulted in some increases in maximal overground walking speed [99].

Activity-based therapies

In the long term, LT will provide a behavioral therapy that independently supports positive outcomes. It may also serve as a catalyst in tandem with electrical stimulation or pharmacologic agents that when combined form an even better response. Already, researchers have explored the combined use of drugs and LT as well FES and LT to advance recovery [100–102]. Thus, a continuum of physical rehabilitation interventions may be considered and categorized as activity-based therapies (Table 1). The

Table 1
Physical rehabilitation interventions that promote recovery of function and/or compensation to regain function

Rehabilitation for mobility					
Activity-based		Activity/compensation		Compensation	
Intervention	Neuromuscular activity	Intervention	Neuromuscular activity	Intervention	Neuromuscular activity
Locomotor training for stepping	Intrinsic below lesion level	Walking with FES for individual movements or joints	Intrinsic below lesion level with extrinsic activation for deficits	Walking with reciprocating gait orthosis (RGO) or long-leg braces	None; bracing and mechanical device for deficits
		Ankle foot orthotic use during walking	Intrinsic below lesion level with bracing for deficits	Power or manual wheelchair	None
		Ambulation with FES implanted electrodes	Extrinsic below lesion level		
Locomotor training for standing	Intrinsic below lesion level	Standing with FES	Extrinsic below lesion level	Standing frame	Minimal
		Standing with braces	Intrinsic below lesion level with bracing replacing function		
Muscle strengthening below lesion level	Intrinsic			Muscle strengthening Above Lesion Level	None
FES cycling	Extrinsic below level of the lesion				
Voluntary cycling	Intrinsic below level of the lesion				

criteria, activity-based versus compensation, intrinsic versus extrinsic activation of the nervous system, and activation of the nervous system below or above the lesion are used to categorize rehabilitation strategies for mobility.

For example, even individuals with clinically complete injury can experience activity-based therapies with manual or robotic assistance and when electrical stimulation is used on muscles below the level of the lesion during stand and step training [97–99,103]. In individuals with incomplete injury, this can also occur with many different interventions (ie, FES cycling?) [104,105] but with a primary aim of facilitating activation of the neuromuscular system below the level of lesion [104,105]. A further consideration is the activation of the nervous system by extrinsic means, such as electrical stimulation, compared with activation intrinsically by the nervous system. An example of intrinsic activation is the increase in leg extensor muscle EMG activity in response to increasing vertical load while standing in both nondisabled persons and persons with complete and incomplete spinal cord injuries [67]. Also important is a distinction between an outcome that achieves a functional goal compared with recovery of a function. Learning to drive a powered wheelchair with a mouthpiece is considered a "functional goal," whereas improving the ability to stand or step is an example of functional recovery of the neuromuscular system.

FES may be a tool to improve standing or stepping. If appropriate sensory information is important for retraining, then can current stimulation parameters be effective in relearning or can future FES stimulation paradigms be incorporated with the intrinsic properties of the spinal cord? Whether FES is used through implanted electrodes or surface stimulation to muscles, recovery of function will be established if the stimulation is no longer needed to perform the task. If the FES remains necessary and the nervous system is quiescent in its absence, then it is likely that FES under those conditions is not contributing to the recovery of function. In this instance, FES is acting in a compensatory role as a neuroprosthesis. Further studies are needed to understand the most optimal approach to retraining the nervous system and to determine the most appropriate use of electrical stimulation in severely impaired individuals.

Strengthening muscles above the level of the lesion is a compensation-based therapy; however, activating and strengthening muscles below the level of the lesion is an activity-based therapy. Whether intrinsically driving [106] or extrinsically activating muscles below the level of the lesion [104,107–110], neuromuscular adaptations result in greater voluntary torque and increased rate of torque production in persons with incomplete and complete SCI. Persistence of such benefits is dependent on the capacity of the individual to continue neural activation within the context of daily function or remain dependent on extrinsic input for activation. Whether FES cycling promotes recovery of muscle activation specific to the task of walking has yet to be determined.

Outcome measures: functional goals and recovery of function

The outcome measures studied are critical to interpreting the effect and clinical meaningfulness of compensation-based and activity-based therapies, including LT. Because physical rehabilitation as an agent for recovery is a new perspective, comparable outcome measures need to be developed that measure recovery. Current clinical measures address the ability to perform a task as a functional goal but may not specifically address recovery of function [25]. A task may be performed using a compensatory strategy or via recovery of the neuromuscular control specific to that task. Achievement of the compensatory behavior is consistent with gaining a new ability to accomplish a goal (eg, use of forearm crutches to bear partial weight while using a head–hip strategy to advance a pair of long-leg braces forward for ambulation), whereas retraining and recovery of function entails regaining the specific function associated with the task (eg, activating limb extension and support for standing and flexor activity for swing).

Clinical outcome measures target achieving the task goal, for example, walking performance [87,111,112]. Outcome measures include walking speed (m/s) at self-selected and fastest speeds (treadmill or overground), time to traverse prescribed distances (50 m walk test), endurance–distance walked in set time, amount of assistance required (ie, braces, assistive device, or physical assistance) (WISCI II) [113,114], ability to negotiate obstacles, and balance ability. The assessment of clinical meaningfulness of an outcome is particularly important. Gait speed, as a continuous variable, may provide the most meaningful outcome relative to the achievement of speeds standard for adults (1.2 m/s) [69] and required for community ambulation for safe street crossing at traffic lights [115–119]. Percent changes in gait speed may be statistically significant but may portray an inflated view of meaningful value. For example, when a 100% improvement in gait speed reflects a change from 0.05 m/s to 0.1 m/s the change may be negligible to the observer and, unfortunately, of little consequence as a behavioral gain. However, a 100% improvement in gait speed from 0.4 to 0.8 m/s may be a meaningful change and reflect a functional shift from household to community ambulator. For gait speed to be a measure of recovery, the variability of the measure and the clinical meaning of improved speed should be established, as well as consider the influence of different assistive devices.

Walking recovery, regaining the specific functions that afford walking capacity, will require new measures reflecting interim, yet, progressive changes across training time. Instruments that measure specific function for walking entail the capacity to produce a reciprocal stepping pattern, balance during propulsion, and adaptation to the environment [39,120]. A single measure is unlikely to reflect the recovery of function of an individual or subpopulations. Composite outcome measures or targeted measures for specific phases of recovery may be more reflective of recovery. Assessing the neuromuscular capacity below the level of lesion may provide a more objective and sensitive assessment during recovery [59–62]. The presence of clonus and spasticity may also now be considered as a positive indication that neural networks are active and have the potential for functional reorganization rather than as a consequence of loss of supraspinal input that prohibits recovery of motor function that should be eliminated by pharmacologic or surgical interventions [121,122].

As the treadmill environment affords a permissive and controlled environment for retraining, it may also offer an environment for assessing the nervous systems' capacity to step, balance, and adapt as well as assessing the recovery of walking specific functions. In this environment, for instance, BWS required to maintain lower limb extension or upright posture may be titrated and quantified indicating increments of capacity and recovery from an initial evaluation through a training process. Incremental gains observed in the training environment are likely to be more sensitive and informative of capacity/recovery when compared with the gains observed by routine clinical measures overground (eg, self-selected gait speed). Thresholds of recovery specific to walking capacity may ultimately correlate with clinical gains overground. For example, a patient demonstrated no significant gains in gait speed overground BWS, and manual assistance had decreased and been eliminated while walking in the BWS environment [46]. Thus, the continual decline in BWS and manual assistance relative to improved control of the trunk, upright posture, and limb flexion during walking can identify changes in recovery before the current outcomes. Other means of measurement may afford greater quantification in this environment and are a critical area of ongoing and future development. Secondary and tertiary benefits of therapy on the ability to perform activities of daily living, health, and quality of life may also be considered as outcome measures [93,94,123].

Clinical decision making for recovery of function

Much of today's research [66,89,124] emphasis is on comparing the effectiveness or benefits of one therapeutic intervention compared with another in sample populations grouped according to AIS classification. Because activity-based therapy aimed at recovery after SCI represents a paradigm shift, our efforts as researchers should parallel this shift of emphasis. The information gained comparing one intervention with another may be insufficient when considering the complexity of SCI and its consequences on walking. The heterogeneity of the SCI population makes the interpretation of findings across the varying studies limited even when the AIS classification is used to categorize injury severity. Although this classification represents neurologic recovery of sensorimotor function based on voluntary control, it may not adequately assess the residual motor capacity specific to the recovery of function or the potential to retrain the spinal networks [125,126]. Interpreting the literature and, more importantly, designing research studies and interventions will require scientists and clinicians to better categorize the impairments and task-specific functional limitations secondary to injury and its consequences.

Programs of therapy will likely differ between two individuals that are both AIS C and that show dramatically different lower extremity and trunk activation patterns [127]. The individual with predominant flexor activity may require load-bearing activity to promote extensor activity during stance. The individual with low levels of activation may benefit from an extrinsic-based approach to increase not only activation but torque production. Additionally, therapies provided acutely may differ from those provided in chronic states after SCI. Combined therapies may be appropriate to activate a flexor pattern in some individuals with this functional deficit yet not appropriate for others. The consistency of repetition by robotic-assist training may provide the intensity necessary to activate or change flexor activity to alternating flexor and extensor activity yet only is the first step in a series of therapeutic steps [85,92,128]. Furthermore, pharmacology may be an adjunct to LT or cycling or other activity-based therapy. As a hybrid therapy, this intervention may provide a timely step toward recovery and constitute an important clinical treatment decision.

Summary

Physical rehabilitation as an agent for recovery reflects a paradigm shift in our expectations after SCI. The shift is from the view of SCI as an event from which one does not recover significant function and thus requires compensation for functional loss and impairment to the view that it is possible to restore function through activity-dependent therapies using intrinsic properties of the nervous system to generate and retrain motor responses. Recovery thus requires retraining of the neuromuscular system to execute a task. Compensation replicates the task by using assistive devices, braces, a wheelchair, or alternative movement patterns to reach a goal that allows the individual to function in their daily lives.

Many studies now support that recovery can be facilitated by physical rehabilitation interventions, and the improvement of neuromuscular function can continue to occur even years after injury. If compensation methods are inconsistent with the functional recovery, then the clinician's challenge is to partner with the patient to determine the best practice guidelines to achieve daily activities of life by regaining lost functions while also continuing to promote the recovery of function. Future studies should be designed to identify the specific patient populations that can most effectively benefit from activity-based therapies and to continue to understand neuroplasticity to improve recovery of function in all patient populations.

A clinical decision-making algorithm for best practice will incorporate therapies, in combination or in sequence, that meet the individual's needs throughout the course of recovery. Recovery will thus entail a program of therapies [129] and not a single therapy to meet the changing needs of the patient as he or she advances on the path to recovery. Current challenges to these advances include classification of a heterogeneous population according to task-specific residual motor control [130], sufficient outcome measures to compare interventions, and the cost to implement rehabilitation clinical trials. Although this review has targeted emerging activity-based therapies for recovery of walking, application of activity-dependent neuroplasticity to other physiologic functions may prove to be valid. The continued partnership of scientists, clinicians, and consumers will advance the agenda forward to consumer priorities for recovery of other important functions after spinal cord injury [131].

References

[1] Consortium for Spinal Cord Medicine. Outcomes following traumatic spinal cord injury: clinical practice guidelines for health-care professionals. Washington, DC: Paralyzed Veterans of America; 1999.

[2] Kirshblum SC, O'Connor KC. Levels of spinal cord injury and predictors of neurologic recovery. Phys Med Rehabil Clin N Am 2000;11:1–27, vii.

[3] Burns SP, Golding DG, Rolle WA Jr, et al. Recovery of ambulation in motor-incomplete tetraplegia. Arch Phys Med Rehabil 1997;78:1169–72.

[4] Crozier KS, Cheng LL, Graziani V, et al. Spinal cord injury: prognosis for ambulation based on quadriceps recovery. Paraplegia 1992;30:762–7.

[5] Burns AS, Ditunno JF. Establishing prognosis and maximizing functional outcomes after spinal cord injury: a review of current and future directions in rehabilitation management. Spine 2001;26:S137–45.

[6] Waters RL, Adkins R, Yakura J, et al. Prediction of ambulatory performance based on motor scores derived from standards of the American Spinal Injury Association. Arch Phys Med Rehabil 1994;75:756–60.

[7] Marino RJ, Barros T, Biering-Sorensen F, et al. International standards for neurological classification of spinal cord injury. J Spinal Cord Med 2003;26(Suppl 1):S50–6.

[8] Waters RL, Adkins RH, Yakura JS, et al. Motor and sensory recovery following complete tetraplegia. Arch Phys Med Rehabil 1993;74:242–7.

[9] Kirshblum S, Millis S, McKinley W, et al. Late neurologic recovery after traumatic spinal cord injury. Arch Phys Med Rehabil 2004;85:1811–7.

[10] Oleson CV, Burns AS, Ditunno JF, et al. Prognostic value of pinprick preservation in motor complete, sensory incomplete spinal cord injury. Arch Phys Med Rehabil 2005;86:988–92.

[11] Ditunno JF Jr, Stover SL, Freed MM, et al. Motor recovery of the upper extremities in traumatic quadriplegia: a multicenter study. Arch Phys Med Rehabil 1992;73:431–6.

[12] Brown PJ, Marino RJ, Herbison GJ, et al. The 72-hour examination as a predictor of recovery in motor complete quadriplegia. Arch Phys Med Rehabil 1991;72:546–8.

[13] Waters RL, Adkins RH, Yakura JS, et al. Motor and sensory recovery following incomplete tetraplegia. Arch Phys Med Rehabil 1994;75:306–11.

[14] Kuhn RA. Functional capacity of the isolated human spinal cord. Brain 1950;73:1–51.

[15] Dietz V. Human neuronal control of automatic functional movements: interaction between central programs and afferent input. Physiol Rev 1992;72:33–69.

[16] Vilensky JA, Gilman S, Dunn EA, et al. Utilization of the Denny-Brown collection: differential recovery of forelimb and hind limb stepping after extensive unilateral cerebral lesions. Behav Brain Res 1997;82:223–33.

[17] Fouad K, Pearson K. Restoring walking after spinal cord injury. Prog Neurobiol 2004;73: 107–26.

[18] Bracken MB. Pharmacological treatment of acute spinal cord injury: current status and future prospects. Paraplegia 1992;30:102–7.
[19] Bracken MB, Shepard MJ, Holford TR, et al. Methylprednisolone or tirilazad mesylate administration after acute spinal cord injury: 1-year follow up. Results of the third National Acute Spinal Cord Injury randomized controlled trial. J Neurosurg 1998;89:699–706.
[20] Geisler FH, Coleman WP, Grieco G, et al. The Sygen multicenter acute spinal cord injury study. Spine 2001;26:S87–98.
[21] Geisler FH, Coleman WP, Grieco G, et al. Measurements and recovery patterns in a multicenter study of acute spinal cord injury. Spine 2001;26:S68–86.
[22] Bracken MB, Shepard MJ, Holford TR, et al. Administration of methylprednisolone for 24 or 48 hours or tirilazad mesylate for 48 hours in the treatment of acute spinal cord injury. Results of the Third National Acute Spinal Cord Injury Randomized Controlled Trial. National Acute Spinal Cord Injury Study. JAMA 1997;277:1597–604.
[23] Dolan EJ, Tator CH, Endrenyi L. The value of decompression for acute experimental spinal cord compression injury. J Neurosurg 1980;53:749–55.
[24] Cotler JM, Herbison GJ, Nasuti JF, et al. Closed reduction of traumatic cervical spine dislocation using traction weights up to 140 pounds. Spine 1993;18:386–90.
[25] Hall KM, Cohen ME, Wright J, et al. Characteristics of the functional independence measure in traumatic spinal cord injury. Arch Phys Med Rehabil 1999;80:1471–6.
[26] National Spinal Cord Injury Statistical Center. Department of Education [Spinal cord injury information network-fact sheet]. Available at: http://www.spinalcord.uab.edu. Accessed March, 2007.
[27] Somers M. Spinal cord injury: functional rehabilitation. London: Prentice-Hall Inc.; 2001.
[28] Atrice MB, Morrison SA, McDowell SL, et al. Traumatic spinal cord injury. In: Umphred DA, editor. Neurological rehabilitation. 5th edition. St. Louis (MO): Mosby Inc.; 2005. p. 605–57.
[29] Fulk G, Schmitz TJ, Behrman AL. Traumatic spinal cord injury. In: O' Sullivan SB, Schmitz TJ, editors. Physical rehabilitation—assessment and treatment. Philadelphia: F.A. Davis Company; 2007. p. 937–98.
[30] Neumann D, Lanouette M. Clinical kinesiology applied to persons with quadriplegia. Milwaukee (WI): Marquette University, Zablocki VA Medical Center; 2002.
[31] Pepin A, Ladouceur M, Barbeau H. Treadmill walking in incomplete spinal-cord-injured subjects: 2. Factors limiting the maximal speed. Spinal Cord 2003;41:271–9.
[32] Pepin A, Norman KE, Barbeau H. Treadmill walking in incomplete spinal-cord-injured subjects: 1. Adaptation to changes in speed. Spinal Cord 2003;41:257–70.
[33] van Hedel HJ, Wirz M, Dietz V. Assessing walking ability in subjects with spinal cord injury: validity and reliability of 3 walking tests. Arch Phys Med Rehabil 2005;86:190–6.
[34] Visintin M, Barbeau H. The effects of parallel bars, body weight support and speed on the modulation of the locomotor pattern of spastic paretic gait. A preliminary communication. Paraplegia 1994;32:540–53.
[35] Ladouceur M, Pepin A, Norman KE, et al. Recovery of walking after spinal cord injury. Adv Neurol 1997;72:249–55.
[36] Brotherton SS, Krause JS, Nietert PJ. Falls in individuals with incomplete spinal cord injury. Spinal Cord 2007;45:37–40.
[37] Leroux A, Fung J, Barbeau H. Postural adaptation to walking on inclined surfaces: II. Strategies following spinal cord injury. Clin Neurophysiol 2006;117:1273–82.
[38] Ladouceur M, Barbeau H, McFadyen BJ. Kinematic adaptations of spinal cord-injured subjects during obstructed walking. Neurorehabil Neural Repair 2003;17:25–31.
[39] Barbeau H. Locomotor training in neurorehabilitation: emerging rehabilitation concepts. Neurorehabil Neural Repair 2003;17:3–11.
[40] Barbeau H, Nadeau S, Garneau C. Physical determinants, emerging concepts, and training approaches in gait of individuals with spinal cord injury. J Neurotrauma 2006;23: 571–85.

[41] Dietz V, Harkema SJ. Locomotor activity in spinal cord-injured persons. J Appl Physiol 2004;96:1954–60.
[42] Edgerton VR, Tillakaratne NJ, Bigbee AJ, et al. Plasticity of the spinal neural circuitry after injury. Annu Rev Neurosci 2004;27:145–67.
[43] Wolpaw JR. Spinal cord plasticity in acquisition and maintenance of motor skills. Acta Physiol (Oxf) 2007;189:155–69.
[44] Edgerton VR, Roy RR, Hodgson JA, et al. A physiological basis for the development of rehabilitative strategies for spinally injured patients. J Am Paraplegia Soc 1991;14:150–7.
[45] Hodgson JA, Roy RR, de Leon R, et al. Can the mammalian lumbar spinal cord learn a motor task? Med Sci Sports Exerc 1994;26:1491–7.
[46] Behrman AL, Lawless-Dixon AR, Davis SB, et al. Locomotor training progression and outcomes after incomplete spinal cord injury. Phys Ther 2005;85:1356–71.
[47] Behrman AL, Harkema SJ. Locomotor training after human spinal cord injury: a series of case studies. Phys Ther 2000;80:688–700.
[48] Rossignol IS, Barbeau H. New approaches to locomotor rehabilitation in spinal cord injury [editorial comment] [see comments]. Ann Neurol 1995;37:555–6.
[49] Norman KE, Pepin A, Ladouceur M, et al. A treadmill apparatus and harness support for evaluation and rehabilitation of gait. Arch Phys Med Rehabil 1995;76:772–8.
[50] Courtney McGrath, Reversing Paralysis. Available at: http://www.kennedykrieger.org/kki_touch_article.jsp?pid=3663. Accessed April, 2007.
[51] Beyond Therapy Program. Available at: http://www.shepherd.org/patcare/spec/beyond.asp. Accessed April, 2007.
[52] NeuroRecovery Network at Christopher and Dana Reeve Foundation. Available at: http://www.christopherreeve.org/atf/cf/{219882E9-DFFF-4CC0-95EE-3A62423C40EC}/nrn%20brochureLATEST.pdf. Accessed April, 2007.
[53] Restorative Therapies Inc. Available at: http://www.restorative-therapies.com/. Accessed April, 2007.
[54] Magee Rehabilitation Hospital Holds Seminar on Activity Based Therapeutic Rehabilitation on June 9. Available at: http://www.mageerehab.org/news/article12003.html. Accessed April, 2007.
[55] Intense Therapy for Motor Recovery Program. Available at: http://www.maryfreebed.com/secondary.aspx?channelpostingid=270. Accessed April, 2007.
[56] Overview of NextSteps Physical Therapy Centers. Available at: http://www.next-steps.org/therapycenters.htm. Accessed April, 2007.
[57] Daniel E. Graves, PhD, Co-Director and William H. Donovan, MD, Co-Director, Texas Model SCI Program. Available at: http://www.bcm.edu/pmr/research/?PMID=5708. Accessed April, 2007.
[58] Wolpaw JR, Tennissen AM. Activity-dependent spinal cord plasticity in health and disease. Annu Rev Neurosci 2001;24:807–43.
[59] McKay WB, Lim HK, Priebe MM, et al. Clinical neurophysiological assessment of residual motor control in post-spinal cord injury paralysis. Neurorehabil Neural Repair 2004;18:144–53.
[60] McKay WB, Lee DC, Lim HK, et al. Neurophysiological examination of the corticospinal system and voluntary motor control in motor-incomplete human spinal cord injury. Exp Brain Res 2005;163:379–87.
[61] Sherwood AM, Dimitrijevic MR, McKay WB. Evidence of subclinical brain influence in clinically complete spinal cord injury: discomplete SCI. J Neurol Sci 1992;110:90–8.
[62] Sherwood AM, Graves DE, Priebe MM. Altered motor control and spasticity after spinal cord injury: subjective and objective assessment. J Rehabil Res Dev 2000;37:41–52.
[63] Wernig A, Muller S, Nanassy A, et al. Laufband therapy based on 'rules of spinal locomotion' is effective in spinal cord injured persons. Eur J Neurosci 1995;7:823–9.
[64] Lovely RG, Gregor RJ, Roy RR, et al. Effects of training on the recovery of full-weight-bearing stepping in the adult spinal cat. Exp Neurol 1986;92:421–35.

[65] Hidler JM. What is next for locomotor-based studies? J Rehabil Res Dev 2005;42: 10–6.
[66] Field-Fote EC, Lindley SD, Sherman AL. Locomotor training approaches for individuals with spinal cord injury: a preliminary report of walking-related outcomes. J Neurol Phys Ther 2005;29:127–37.
[67] Harkema SJ, Hurley SL, Patel UK, et al. Human lumbosacral spinal cord interprets loading during stepping. J Neurophysiol 1997;77:797–811.
[68] Dietz V, Muller R, Colombo G. Locomotor activity in spinal man: significance of afferent input from joint and load receptors. Brain 2002;125:2626–34.
[69] Craik R, Dutterer L. Spatial and temporal characteristics of foot fall patterns. In: Craik R, Oatis C, editors. Gait analysis: theory and application. St. Louis (MO): Mosby-Year Book; 1995. p. 143–58.
[70] Thomas SL, Gorassini MA. Increases in corticospinal tract function by treadmill training after incomplete spinal cord injury. J Neurophysiol 2005;94:2844–55.
[71] Beres-Jones JA, Harkema SJ. The human spinal cord interprets velocity-dependent afferent input during stepping. Brain 2004;127:2232–46.
[72] Lunenburger L, Bolliger M, Czell D, et al. Modulation of locomotor activity in complete spinal cord injury. Exp Brain Res 2006;174:638–46.
[73] Duysens J, Pearson KG. Inhibition of flexor burst generation by loading ankle extensor muscles in walking cats. Brain Res 1980;187:321–32.
[74] Duysens J, Clarac F, Cruse H. Load-regulating mechanisms in gait and posture: comparative aspects. Physiol Rev 2000;80.83–133.
[75] Ferris DP, Huang HJ, Kao PC. Moving the arms to activate the legs. Exerc Sport Sci Rev 2006;34:113–20.
[76] Barbeau H, Wainberg M, Finch L. Description and application of a system for locomotor rehabilitation. Med Biol Eng Comput 1987;25:341–4.
[77] Finch L, Barbeau H, Arsenault B. Influence of body weight support on normal human gait: development of a gait retraining strategy. Phys Ther 1991;71:842–55 [discussion: 855–6].
[78] Chen G, Patten C. Treadmill training with harness support: selection of parameters for individuals with poststroke hemiparesis. J Rehabil Res Dev 2006;43:485–98.
[79] Krassioukov AV, Harkema SJ. Effect of harness application and postural changes on cardiovascular parameters of individuals with spinal cord injury. Spinal Cord 2006;44: 780–6.
[80] Frey M, Colombo G, Vaglio M, et al. A novel mechatronic body weight support system. IEEE Trans Neural Syst Rehabil Eng 2006;14:311–21.
[81] Martin J, Plummer P, Bowden MG, et al. Body weight support systems: considerations for clinicians. Phys Ther Rev 2006;11:143–52.
[82] Wernig A, Muller S. Laufband locomotion with body weight support improved walking in persons with severe spinal cord injuries. Paraplegia 1992;30:229–38.
[83] Colombo G, Wirz M, Dietz V. Driven gait orthosis for improvement of locomotor training in paraplegic patients. Spinal Cord 2001;39:252–5.
[84] Colombo G, Joerg M, Schreier R, et al. Treadmill training of paraplegic patients using a robotic orthosis. J Rehabil Res Dev 2000;37:693–700.
[85] Hornby TG, Zemon DH, Campbell D. Robotic-assisted, body-weight-supported treadmill training in individuals following motor incomplete spinal cord injury. Phys Ther 2005;85: 52–66.
[86] Hidler JM, Wall AE. Alterations in muscle activation patterns during robotic-assisted walking. Clin Biomech (Bristol, Avon) 2005;20:184–93.
[87] Behrman AL, Bowden MG, Nair PM. Neuroplasticity after spinal cord injury and training: an emerging paradigm shift in rehabilitation and walking recovery. Phys Ther 2006;86: 1406–25.
[88] Dobkin BH, Apple D, Barbeau H, et al. Methods for a randomized trial of weight-supported treadmill training versus conventional training for walking during inpatient

rehabilitation after incomplete traumatic spinal cord injury. Neurorehabil Neural Repair 2003;17:153–67.

[89] Dobkin B, Apple D, Barbeau H, et al. Weight-supported treadmill vs over-ground training for walking after acute incomplete SCI. Neurology 2006;66:484–93.

[90] Field-Fote EC, Tepavac D. Improved intralimb coordination in people with incomplete spinal cord injury following training with body weight support and electrical stimulation. Phus Ther 2002;82:707–15.

[91] Field-Fote EC. Combined use of body weight support, functional electric stimulation, and treadmill training to improve walking ability in individuals with chronic incomplete spinal cord injury. Arch Phys Med Rehabil 2001;82:818–24.

[92] Wirz M, Zemon DH, Rupp R, et al. Effectiveness of automated locomotor training in patients with chronic incomplete spinal cord injury: a multicenter trial. Arch Phys Med Rehabil 2005;86:672–80.

[93] Hicks AL, Adams MM, Martin Ginis K, et al. Long-term body-weight-supported treadmill training and subsequent follow-up in persons with chronic SCI: effects on functional walking ability and measures of subjective well-being. Spinal Cord 2005;43: 291–8.

[94] Effing TW, van Meeteren NL, van Asbeck FW, et al. Body weight-supported treadmill training in chronic incomplete spinal cord injury: a pilot study evaluating functional health status and quality of life. Spinal Cord 2006;44:287–96.

[95] Dietz V, Wirz M, Curt A, et al. Locomotor pattern in paraplegic patients: training effects and recovery of spinal cord function. Spinal Cord 1998;36:380–90.

[96] Fung J, Barbeau H. Effects of conditioning cutaneomuscular stimulation on the soleus H-reflex in normal and spastic paretic subjects during walking and standing. J Neurophysiol 1994;72:2090–104.

[97] Ladouceur M, Barbeau H. Functional electrical stimulation-assisted walking for persons with incomplete spinal injuries: longitudinal changes in maximal overground walking speed. Scand J Rehabil Med 2000;32:28–36.

[98] Ladouceur M, Barbeau H. Functional electrical stimulation-assisted walking for persons with incomplete spinal injuries: changes in the kinematics and physiological cost of overground walking. Scand J Rehabil Med 2000;32:72–9.

[99] Barbeau H, Ladouceur M, Mirbagheri MM, et al. The effect of locomotor training combined with functional electrical stimulation in chronic spinal cord injured subjects: walking and reflex studies. Brain Res Rev 2002;40:274–91.

[100] Norman KE, Pepin A, Barbeau H. Effects of drugs on walking after spinal cord injury. Spinal Cord 1998;36:699–715.

[101] Rossignol S, Barbeau H. Pharmacology of locomotion: an account of studies in spinal cats and spinal cord injured subjects. J Am Paraplegia Soc 1993;16:190–6.

[102] Fung J, Stewart JE, Barbeau H. The combined effects of clonidine and cyproheptadine with interactive training on the modulation of locomotion in spinal cord injured subjects. J Neurol Sci 1990;100:85–93.

[103] Postans NJ, Hasler JP, Granat MH, et al. Functional electric stimulation to augment partial weight-bearing supported treadmill training for patients with acute incomplete spinal cord injury: a pilot study. Arch Phys Med Rehabil 2004;85:604–10.

[104] Scremin AM, Kurta L, Gentili A, et al. Increasing muscle mass in spinal cord injured persons with a functional electrical stimulation exercise program. Arch Phys Med Rehabil 1999;80:1531–6.

[105] Donaldson N, Perkins TA, Fitzwater R, et al. FES cycling may promote recovery of leg function after incomplete spinal cord injury. Spinal Cord 2000;38:680–2.

[106] Gregory CM, Bowden MG, Jayaraman A, et al. Resistance training and locomotor recovery after incomplete spinal cord injury: a case series. Spinal Cord 2007 Jan 16; [Epub ahead of print].

[107] Sabatier MJ, Stoner L, Mahoney ET, et al. Electrically stimulated resistance training in SCI individuals increases muscle fatigue resistance but not femoral artery size or blood flow. Spinal Cord 2006;44:227–33.
[108] Mahoney ET, Bickel CS, Elder C, et al. Changes in skeletal muscle size and glucose tolerance with electrically stimulated resistance training in subjects with chronic spinal cord injury. Arch Phys Med Rehabil 2005;86:1502–4.
[109] Shields RK, Dudley-Javoroski S. Musculoskeletal plasticity after acute spinal cord injury: effects of long-term neuromuscular electrical stimulation training. J Neurophysiol 2006;95: 2380–90.
[110] Ragnarsson KT. Physiological effects of functional electrical stimulation-induced exercises in spinal cord-injured individuals. Clin Orthop Relat Res 1988;53–63.
[111] Dobkin B, Barbeau H, Deforge D, et al. The evolution of walking-related outcomes over the first 12 weeks of rehabilitation for incomplete traumatic spinal cord injury: the multicenter randomized Spinal Cord Injury Locomotor Trial. Neurorehabil Neural Repair 2007;21: 25–35.
[112] Steeves JD, Lammertse D, Curt A, et al. Guidelines for the conduct of clinical trials for spinal cord injury (SCI) as developed by the ICCP panel: clinical trial outcome measures. Spinal Cord 2007 Mar;45(3):190–205.
[113] Dittuno PL, Dittuno JF Jr. Walking index for spinal cord injury (WISCI II): scale revision. Spinal Cord 2001;39:654–656.
[114] Ditunno JF Jr, Ditunno PL, Graziani V, et al. Walking index for spinal cord injury (WISCI): an international multicenter validity and reliability study. Spinal Cord 2000;38:234–43.
[115] Lerner-Frankiel MB, Varcas S, Brown MB, et al. Functional community ambulation: what are your criteria? Clin Manage Phys Ther 1986;6:12–5.
[116] Shumway-Cook A, Patla A, Stewart A, et al. Environmental components of mobility disability in community-living older persons. J Am Geriatr Soc 2003;51:393–8.
[117] Patla AE, Shumway-Cook A. Dimensions of mobility: defining the complexity and difficulty associated with community mobility. Journal of Aging and Physical Activity 1999;7:7–19.
[118] Langlois JA, Keyl PM, Guralnik JM, et al. Characteristics of older pedestrians who have difficulty crossing the street. Am J Public Health 1997;87:393–7.
[119] Perry J, Garrett M, Gronley JK, et al. Classification of walking handicap in the stroke population. Stroke 1995;26:982–9.
[120] Forssberg H. Spinal locomotor functions and descending control. In: Sjolund B, Bjorklund RA, editors. Brainstem control of spinal mechanisms. Amsterdam: Elsevier Biomedical; 1982. p. 253–71.
[121] Dietz V. Neurophysiology of gait disorders: present and future applications. Electroencephalogr Clin Neurophysiol 1997;103:333–55.
[122] Beres-Jones JA, Johnson TD, Harkema SJ. Clonus after human spinal cord injury cannot be attributed solely to recurrent muscle-tendon stretch. Exp Brain Res 2003;149:222–36.
[123] Martin Ginis KA, Latimer AE. The effects of single bouts of body-weight supported treadmill training on the feeling states of people with spinal cord injury. Spinal Cord 2007;45: 112–5.
[124] Protas EJ, Holmes SA, Qureshy H, et al. Supported treadmill ambulation training after spinal cord injury: a pilot study. Arch Phys Med Rehabil 2001;82:825–31.
[125] Dimitrijevic MR. Residual motor functions in spinal cord injury. Adv Neurol 1988;47: 138–55.
[126] Kern H, McKay WB, Dimitrijevic MM, et al. Motor control in the human spinal cord and the repair of cord function. Curr Pharm Des 2005;11:1429–39.
[127] Maegele M, Muller S, Wernig A, et al. Recruitment of spinal motor pools during voluntary movements versus stepping after human spinal cord injury. J Neurotrauma 2002;19: 1217–29.

[128] Israel JF, Campbell DD, Kahn JH, et al. Metabolic costs and muscle activity patterns during robotic- and therapist-assisted treadmill walking in individuals with incomplete spinal cord injury. Phys Ther 2006;86:1466–78.

[129] Teng YD, Liao W, Choi H, et al. Physical activity-mediated functional recovery after spinal cord injury: potential roles of neural stem cells. Regenerative Medicine 2006;1:763–76.

[130] Norton JA, Gorassini MA. Changes in cortically related intermuscular coherence accompanying improvements in locomotor skills in incomplete spinal cord injury. J Neurophysiol 2006;95:2580–9.

[131] Anderson KD. Targeting recovery: priorities of the spinal cord-injured population. J Neurotrauma 2004;21:1371–83.

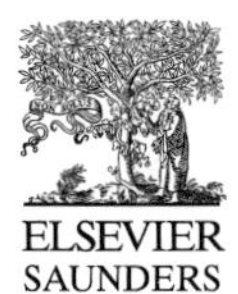
ELSEVIER
SAUNDERS

Phys Med Rehabil Clin N Am
18 (2007) 203–216

PHYSICAL MEDICINE
AND REHABILITATION
CLINICS OF
NORTH AMERICA

Acute Respiratory Infections in Persons with Spinal Cord Injury

Stephen P. Burns, MD[a,b,c,*]

[a]*Spinal Cord Injury Service (128), VA Puget Sound Health Care System, 1660 S. Columbian Way, Seattle, WA 98108, USA*
[b]*Department of Rehabilitation Medicine, Box 356490, University of Washington, Seattle, WA 98195, USA*
[c]*Harborview Injury Prevention and Research Center, 325 Ninth Avenue, Box 359960, Seattle, WA 98104, USA*

Morbidity and mortality caused by respiratory infections

Respiratory disorders are the leading cause of death in persons with both acute and chronic spinal cord injury (SCI). Pneumonia occurs in 50% of patients with acute tetraplegia during acute hospitalization and rehabilitation [1]. Respiratory disorders account for 28% of deaths in the first year after injury and 22% of deaths in later years [2]. In patients who survive for at least 24 hours after injury, pneumonia or influenza causes 16.5% of all deaths [3]. This contrasts with that of the general population of the United States, for which pneumonia and influenza account for only 2.5% of deaths and the two diseases in combination are the eighth leading cause of death [4]. The standardized mortality ratio, a measure that adjusts for age, sex, and race, indicates that the rate of fatal pneumonia is elevated by a factor of 37 for people with SCI; persons with complete tetraplegia die from pneumonia at a rate that is 150 times higher than a matched population without SCI [2].

Respiratory disorders are also a leading cause of rehospitalization after SCI [5]. Based on United States (US) Model SCI Systems (MSCIS) data,

This article represents the opinion of the authors and does not necessarily represent the Department of Veterans Affairs.

This work was supported by the Department of Veterans Affairs and Grant No. R49 CCR002570-19 from the Centers for Disease Control and Prevention.

* Spinal Cord Injury Service (128), VA Puget Sound Health Care System, 1660 S. Columbian Way, Seattle, WA 98108.

E-mail address: spburns@u.washington.edu

doi:10.1016/j.pmr.2007.02.001 *pmr.theclinics.com*

they are the third most common reason for hospitalization during the first year after SCI. A population-based study from Alberta, Canada found respiratory complications to be the leading cause of rehospitalization during the first 6 years after injury [6]. For patients with C1 to C4 American Spinal Injury Association (ASIA) Impairment Scale A-C tetraplegia, they account for 30% of rehopitalizations across all years of follow-up [5].

In spite of the importance of respiratory infections as a cause of death in persons with SCI, few studies have examined the topic. The majority have reported on the incidence of respiratory complications during acute care and rehabilitation, in settings such as the MSCIS hospitals. Rehospitalization rates and causes of death in persons with chronic SCI have also been published using data from the US MSCIS as well as from other nations. More recently, data on outpatient respiratory infections in Veterans Affairs (VA) patients with SCI have been reported. The populations included in these studies may not be representative of all persons with SCI. Most have focused on epidemiologic aspects of respiratory infections. There remains a need to conduct clinical trials of preventive measures and treatments to reduce the morbidity and mortality associated with respiratory infections in this population.

Predisposing factors for persons with spinal cord injury

SCI can cause multiple alterations in normal physiology that may increase the likelihood of the development of respiratory infections (incidence) or increase the chance of dying from an infection (case fatality). The most obvious of these dysfunctions caused by SCI is weakness of the respiratory muscles. If the neurologic level is at C5 or rostral, there may be some degree of diaphragm weakness or even complete paralysis with higher level motor-complete injuries. At lower neurologic levels, diaphragm innervation is intact, and this normally is sufficient to maintain at least 60% of the predicted vital capacity. Ventilatory failure caused by inspiratory muscle weakness can occur immediately after injury or develop over the first week after the injury. Patients who require mechanical ventilation are susceptible to ventilator-associated pneumonia (VAP). Over the first weeks to months after injury, many patients with partially intact diaphragm innervation acquire the ability to spontaneously ventilate, which is in part caused by strength recovery in the diaphragm. Approximately 7% of persons with SCI will be ventilator dependent when discharged from rehabilitation [7]. Patients with reduced inspiratory muscle strength are predisposed to microatelectasis, which may promote the development of pneumonia in atelectatic segments of the lung.

Severe expiratory muscle weakness is more prevalent in persons with SCI and is likely the most important factor increasing the incidence and case fatality for pneumonia. Expiratory muscle weakness, resulting in low voluntary cough peak expiratory flow, is strongly associated with unsuccessful extubation and increased in-hospital mortality in the general population [8]. Because the primary expiratory muscles, the internal intercostals and abdominals, have thoracic innervation, they will be paralyzed completely in all patients with motor-complete tetraplegia. Expiratory strength increases incrementally with each additional neurologic level and is essentially normal at the T12 neurologic level and below; therefore, patients with high-level paraplegia have a similar degree of weakness to those with low-level tetraplegia. The main consequence of expiratory muscle weakness is a reduced peak cough flow, which is ineffective for clearance of bronchial secretions. With a peak cough flow of less than 2.7 L/sec (160 L/min), there is inadequate airflow to mobilize secretions out of the bronchi and trachea [9]. To compensate for weak cough strength, aggressive multimodal respiratory therapy interventions are required for secretion mobilization [10]. Measures to promote secretion mobilization are listed in Table 1.

Other than respiratory muscle weakness, additional factors predispose patients to respiratory complications. Reduced sympathetic innervation to the lungs occurs with injuries above the mid-thoracic level. The unopposed vagal parasympathetic input in patients with tetraplegia leads to bronchoconstriction and increased bronchial mucus secretion [11]. In patients with acute tetraplegia, bronchial mucus production may exceed 1 L per day, and the secretions are often tenacious, likely because of an altered

Table 1
Secretion mobilization techniques

- Manually-assisted coughing ("quad coughing").
  - Insufflation using bag-valve-mask (eg, AmbuBag) or glossopharyngeal breathing before quad coughing will increase the peak cough flow.
  - Contraindications: inferior vena caval filter, recent abdominal surgery, rib fractures.
- Mechanical insufflation-exsufflation (CoughAssist; J.H. Emerson Co.; Cambridge, MA; www.coughassist.com).
  - Contraindications: bullous emphysema, susceptibility to pneumothorax or pneumomediastinum, or recent barotraumas.
  - Effective cough at inspiratory/expiratory pressures of + 40/−40 cm H_2O; for patient using device for first time, begin with pressures of 15 cm H_2O to familiarize patient with procedure.
  - Typical cough settings: 3 second inhalation phase, 2 second exhalation phase, then pause for 5 seconds.
  - Perform cycle of 4 or 5 assisted coughs, then rest (spontaneously breathing or back on mechanical ventilator) for 30 seconds. Repeat cycle of coughs and rest up to 6 times as needed. Monitor patient symptoms, oxygen saturation, and secretions retrieved to determine when to terminate treatment.
- Percussion (manual percussion; hand-held mechanical percussor).
- Postural drainage.
- Suctioning.
- Bronchoscopy.
- Intrapulmonary percussive ventilation.
- High-frequency chest wall oscillation (The Vest™; Hill-Rom, Inc.; Batesville, Indiana).
- Inhaled mucolytics or hydrating agents for thick, tenacious secretions.

macromolecular composition [12]. Aspiration is relatively common in patients with acute tetraplegia, especially those with predisposing factors such as mechanical ventilation, tracheostomy, anterior neck surgery, or brain injury [13]. Autonomically mediated dynamic dysfunction of the pharynx and upper esophageal sphincter may be an additional contributing factor [14]. In patients with chronic SCI, normal bacterial flora is altered for a number of reasons, including frequent treatment with antibiotics, autonomically mediated changes to the skin, or residence in health care settings, resulting in increased colonization with gram-negative and antibiotic-resistant organisms.

Subclinical adrenal insufficiency is common in this population, and this may blunt the response to sepsis once an infection is present. A diminished immune response in persons with tetraplegia has also been described, which could increase the susceptibility to infection [15]. However, the antibody responses to both pneumococcal and influenza vaccinations in persons with SCI are similar to those in the general population [16,17].

Respiratory infections in outpatients

Pneumonia in the general population

Pneumonia is an acute infection of the pulmonary parenchyma, diagnosed by the presence of symptoms and either an infiltrate on chest radiograph or examination findings indicating consolidation. The most common and most widely studied epidemiologic category of pneumonia is termed *community-acquired pneumonia* (CAP). The most common CAP pathogen overall, as well as for fatal cases alone, is *Streptococcus pneumoniae* (pneumococcus). Other common pathogens include *Hemophilus influenzae*, *Mycoplasma pneumonia*, and *Chlamydophila pneumoniae*. Common risk factors for CAP include young or advanced age, medical comorbidities including chronic lung disease, smoking, immunosuppression, and alcoholism. Use of gastric acid-suppressive drugs (proton pump inhibitors and H2 blockers) also appears to be a risk factor for CAP [18].

Chest radiography is the primary test for establishing the diagnosis of CAP and distinguishing it from acute bronchitis. For patients who are hospitalized, it is recommended that they also have the following tests: complete blood count and differential, serum chemistry panel, liver function tests, oxygen saturation, and blood cultures [19]. A sputum gram stain and culture has also been recommended, but its utility has been debated. A good-quality sputum with a predominant organism can only be obtained in 14% of patients. However, the presence of gram-positive diplococci on Gram stain is highly specific (98%) for pneumococcus [20].

Case fatality for CAP varies widely across studies with varying patient populations. Population-based data on patients receiving care in any setting (inpatient or outpatient) indicate a 1.5% to 2.3% mortality rate, whereas cohort studies indicate a 5.2% mortality rate [21,22]. The Pneumonia Patient Outcome Research Team (Pneumonia PORT) derived an algorithm for determining whether adults with CAP should be hospitalized or treated in the community, based on short-term mortality risk [22]. Patients are stratified into five severity classes, and outpatient treatment is generally recommended for the two lowest risk classes. To qualify for the lowest risk class, an adult would be age 50 years or less, have none of the important comorbidities (cancer, liver disease, congestive heart failure, renal disease, or cerebrovascular disease), have normal mental status, and have normal or only mildly abnormal vital signs. Patients in the two lowest risk categories are anticipated to have a short-term mortality risk of 0.5% or less. The rule is not meant to supersede clinical judgment, nor does it take into account other reasons for hospitalization besides the predicted risk of death from pneumonia. These could include the risk for other adverse events, the availability of support at home, and the likelihood of adherence to therapy and follow-up recommendations.

More recently, it has been recognized that specific outpatient populations with pneumonia are at increased risk for the same highly resistant bacterial pathogens that occur in hospitalized patients. In such cases, the pneumonia is more correctly defined as a health care–associated pneumonia (HCAP), rather than CAP [23]. Risk factors for HCAP include the following: 2 or more days of acute care hospitalization in the prior 90 days; antibiotic therapy, chemotherapy, or wound care in the prior 30 days; residence in a nursing home or long-term care facility; or hemodialysis at a hospital or clinic. The etiologic pathogens in this population as well as treatment principles are thought to be similar to hospital-acquired pneumonia (HAP; see below).

Pneumonia in outpatients with spinal cord injury

Excess mortality caused by an acute condition in a specific population, as with pneumonia in persons with SCI, can be attributable to an increased incidence of the disorder, an increased case fatality when the disorder does develop, or a combination of both factors. There is limited evidence to support both an increased incidence and increased case fatality for pneumonia in persons with chronic SCI. The primary evidence comes from epidemiologic studies that used VA administrative data for persons with SCI.

Smith and colleagues [24] determined outpatient visit rates for acute respiratory infections including pneumonia, based on administrative data for more than 8700 respiratory-related visits by a population of over 13,000 veterans with SCI. Annual outpatient visits for either pneumonia or influenza (nearly all of which were for pneumonia) averaged 29 to 35 per 1000 veterans. A smaller population-based study from Alberta, Canada [6] reported a similar rate of 46 episodes of pneumonia per 1000 patients per year, during the first 6 years after injury. Comparable data for the overall US population indicate a rate of 10 cases of pneumonia per 1000 patients per year.

Using the same VA administrative data as in the study by Weaver and colleagues [25], the outcomes for pneumonia were estimated by determining hospitalization rates and all-cause mortality within 60 days of the visit. After outpatient visits for pneumonia, 46% of patients were hospitalized on the same day, and overall 7.9% of patients died within 60 days of the outpatient visit. By comparison, roughly 25% of the general population with pneumonia will be hospitalized for management [21]. Because the VA study used administrative data, the link between pneumonia diagnosis and subsequent death was not clearly established. However, the case fatality appears to be much higher than the previously cited 1.5% to 2.3% case fatality seen in the general population [21].

Etiologic pathogens for CAP have also been examined using VA administrative data for all SCI veterans hospitalized for treatment of CAP during a 2-year period [26]. The authors also determined whether identification of a causative pathogen for CAP was associated with outcomes in persons with SCI. Cases were identified as CAP if the hospital admission was preceded immediately by outpatient care with a diagnostic code for pneumonia. No significant association was found between the identification of a specific pathogen and mortality in 260 hospitalized SCI patients with CAP. The mean length of stay was 13.5 days, and the overall case fatality was 8.5%.

In that study, a causative pathogen was identified in 24% of cases, with pneumococcus the leading cause of pneumonia (32% of cases), as is true for the general population with CAP. *Pseudomonas*, which is an uncommon pathogen for CAP in the general population, was the second most commonly identified pathogen, occurring in 21% of cases. This finding should prompt clinicians to consider whether their patient with pneumonia has risk factors for HCAP rather than CAP. *Pseudomonas* colonization of the perineum, lower urinary tract, and urine collection system is common in persons with SCI and may be a risk factor for *Pseudomonas* pneumonia in this population [27]. More well-recognized risk factors for gram-negative pneumonia, such as antibiotic treatment or hospitalization in the prior 30 days, pulmonary comorbidity, or aspiration [28], are relatively common in this population as well. In the general population, the relative risk of death is elevated by a factor of 2.6 to 6.4 with *Pseudomonas* pneumonia when compared with other pathogens [29].

An additional VA study characterized the clinical management of CAP at three VA hospitals with specialized SCI services [30]. It used abstraction of individual electronic medical records for SCI veterans who received outpatient or inpatient treatment of CAP during the study period. Cases were identified initially from VA administrative databases using the same method used by Chang and coauthors [26], with the addition of cases that solely received an outpatient diagnosis of pneumonia but did not require hospitalization. Medical records were then reviewed to confirm the diagnosis of CAP, and detailed information on clinical presentation, diagnostic evaluation, and treatments were abstracted from the records. Of the 41 patients,

32 (78%) were hospitalized and only 9 (22%) were treated as outpatients. Because these patients were treated at hospitals with specialized SCI services, this may indicate that SCI specialists are more likely to recommend admission for treatment of HAP. The mean length of stay for hospitalized patients was 19.7 days. The antibiotic coverage received was in accordance with recommendations from the Infectious Disease Society of America for only one half of the patients [19]. After accounting for the relatively high rate of fluoroquinolone resistance at the participating institutions, only 24% of patients received reliable antipseudomonal coverage. The in-hospital mortality rate was 7.3%, and after 3 years of follow-up, 42.1% of hospitalization survivors had died.

General population studies have been used to develop CAP treatment algorithms, involving decisions whether to hospitalize the patient and choice of empiric antibiotic coverage for the most common pathogens. Unfortunately, it is not clear which of these principles may be directly applied to the population with SCI residing in the community. For example, the Pneumonia PORT algorithm assigns no increased risk for either expiratory dysfunction or marginal ventilatory status that may be present because of SCI [22]. Its use is not recommended for persons with SCI, because it is likely to underestimate mortality risk. Recommendations for management of CAP in persons with SCI are summarized in Table 2.

Table 2
Recommendations for management of CAP in persons with SCI

Hospitalization versus Outpatient Treatment:
- Criteria derived from non-SCI population (Pneumonia PORT) may not accurately predict mortality in persons with SCI.
- Hospitalization is strongly encouraged because of high case fatality, likelihood of resistant organisms, and possibility of inadequate secretion mobilization.
- Consider the assistance available at home, the skill of the patient or caregivers with secretion mobilization, the likelihood of compliance with therapy, and the availability and accessibility of follow-up care.

Optimize secretion mobilization:
- Multimodal treatment
- "Quad coughing" (manually assisted coughing); may precede with insufflation.
- Mechanical insufflator-exsufflator (CoughAssist).

Sputum Gram stain and culture.
- Low diagnostic yield but should strongly be considered.
- Could identify an unsuspected highly resistant organism.
- If a low virulence organism is identified, the antibiotic spectrum may be narrowed to avoid promoting antibiotic resistance.

Antibiotics
- Evaluate risk factors for resistant organisms. Should this be considered HCAP?
- Consider empiric antipseudomonal coverage.
- Prompt administration of antibiotics.

Upper respiratory infections and acute bronchitis

Given the high incidence and case fatality seen with pneumonia in outpatients with SCI, the importance of seemingly benign and self-limited conditions as viral upper respiratory infections (URI) and acute bronchitis is not self evident. Both categories of respiratory infections are exceedingly common in the general population. Although they frequently present to primary care settings for evaluation and cause much absenteeism from work and school, they are not generally recognized as causes of morbidity and mortality, with the exception of epidemic influenza A.

However, viral respiratory infections commonly precede or precipitate hospitalizations, especially in patients with chronic underlying pulmonary conditions. Nearly 45% of patients hospitalized with acute respiratory conditions have evidence of recent respiratory tract viral infections [31]. Viruses include those commonly associated with more severe respiratory infections, such as influenza and respiratory syncytial virus but also those associated with the common cold, such as rhinoviruses and coronaviruses [32,33]. In ventilator-dependent patients with neuromuscular disorders, more than 90% of pneumonias and hospitalizations are preceded by upper respiratory tract infections [34].

Upper respiratory infections are primarily viral in etiology. Approximately 10% of pharyngitis cases involves group A *Streptococcus*. The inflammatory response is initially localized to a primary level of the respiratory tract, but in some cases there is spread to adjacent, deeper portions as well. With involvement of the trachea, cough and sputum production can be significant, and symptoms may last for up to 2 weeks. Acute bronchitis indicates an acute respiratory infection involving lower portions of the respiratory tract, with cough as the predominant feature, with or without sputum production. The incidence of acute bronchitis in the general population is about 5%, and up to 90% will seek medical attention. In those without underlying medical conditions, the disorder is usually self-limited with almost no associated mortality, and the key component of evaluation is to rule out more serious conditions such as pneumonia. Because more than 90% of cases are caused by nonbacterial pathogens, routine antibiotic treatment is not recommended [35].

There are limited data to support increased mortality in patients with SCI after acute bronchitis [24]. Based on VA administrative data, veterans with SCI are evaluated in outpatient settings at rates of 26 to 33 visits per year per 1000 veterans for lower respiratory infections (98% of which was acute bronchitis) and 72 to 75 visits per year per 1000 veterans for upper respiratory infections. The mortality rate during the 60 days after the visit was 1.6% for acute bronchitis and 0.7% for upper respiratory tract infections. Only 3.5% of patients seen for acute bronchitis were hospitalized on the day of their outpatient visit; however, 21.9% required hospitalization during the subsequent 60 days. These findings indicate that for persons with SCI, acute bronchitis is associated with a small increase in mortality, and that hospitalization is relatively common after an outpatient evaluation for bronchitis. The study design precluded determining whether pneumonia was misdiagnosed as acute bronchitis in any of these patients or whether pneumonia subsequently developed as a consequence of retained excess bronchial secretions.

Prevention of respiratory infections in outpatients with spinal cord injury

Although respiratory infections are an important source of morbidity and mortality in persons with SCI, it is challenging to conduct prospective research on preventive strategies. Because of the lack of research in this population, the recommendations for prevention are primarily derived from other patient populations, knowledge of pathophysiologic alterations that follow SCI, and clinical experience managing patients who are at high risk for severe respiratory infections.

Influenza vaccine reduces influenza-related hospitalizations, deaths, and secondary complications in elderly patients with and without high-risk medical conditions such as diabetes. Currently, the Centers for Disease Control and Prevention (CDC) recommend annual influenza vaccination for other groups at risk for severe complications from influenza, including those with chronic pulmonary or vascular diseases and residents of chronic care facilities [36]. In 2005, the CDC extended the recommendation to include children and adults with SCI [37].

Pneumococcus is the leading cause of CAP for both the general population and persons with SCI. Pneumococcal polysaccharide vaccine has been shown to reduce the risk of invasive (ie, bacteremic) pneumococcal disease and is considered cost effective for elderly persons. It is also recommended for persons aged 2 years or older who have chronic illnesses including pulmonary diseases [38]. Based on these recommendations, it is routinely offered to persons with SCI, the majority of who have some degree of respiratory impairment. However, only a minority of pneumococcal pneumonias result in bacteremia. The vaccine has not been found to be effective for noninvasive disease, and in elderly patients the rate of CAP and pneumonia hospitalization is unaffected by pneumococcal vaccination [39].

Aggressive mobilization of secretions could play an important role in reducing respiratory infections in outpatients with SCI. A small proportion of patients, primarily those with cervical level injuries, appear to benefit from routine bronchial secretion clearance even in the absence of an acute respiratory infection. This typically can be achieved using quad coughing or mechanical insufflation-exsufflation on a daily basis. More commonly, assistance for secretion mobilization only becomes necessary when a respiratory infection develops. As noted earlier, viral upper respiratory infections or acute bronchitis may lead to subsequent development of pneumonia. Prompt clearance of bronchial secretions may prevent formation of microatelectasis, an increasing bacterial load in the lower respiratory tract, and the development of pneumonia.

Hospital-acquired respiratory infections

Hospital-acquired pneumonia in the general population

HAP is defined as pneumonia occurring 48 hours or more after hospital admission that was not incubating at the time of admission [23]. The rate of HAP in the general population is 5 to 15 per 1000 hospital admissions, and it is the leading cause of death for all hospital-acquired infections. Most findings on HAP have been derived from patients with ventilator-associated pneumonia (VAP), because the risk of pneumonia is 6 to 20 times greater than in nonventilated patients. Risk factors for HAP in the general population include prolonged hospitalization, malnutrition, respiratory failure, sedating medications, dysphagia, central nervous system disorders, supine position during feeding, chronic obstructive pulmonary disease, and the prolonged use of antibiotics [23]. The case fatality rate for HAP may be as high as 70% in certain subpopulations, such as mechanically ventilated patients, although only one third to one half of these deaths are directly attributable to the infection [23].

The most common HAP pathogens include aerobic gram-negative rods such as *Pseudomonas aeruginosa*, *Escherichia coli*, *Klebsiella*, and *Acinetobacter*, as well as gram-positive cocci, with an increasing rate of methicillin-resistant *Staphylococcus aureus*. The spectrum of pathogens is similar for elderly residents of long-term care facilities who have HCAP. The sources of the multidrug-resistant pathogens include health care devices (especially respiratory care equipment), other fomites in the hospital environment, and other patients, and the pathogens are transferred to the patient during routine care. Bacteria may then reach the lower respiratory tract through gross or microscopic aspiration, inhalation, or direct inoculation by respiratory care equipment.

Guidelines on the management and prevention of HAP have been published by the American Thoracic Society, the Infectious Disease Society of America, and the Centers for Disease Control and Prevention [23,40]. Selected recommendations from these documents are summarized in Table 3. As noted earlier, the etiologic pathogens for HCAP are similar to HAP, and most of the HAP management principles are thought to apply to HCAP as well.

Hospital-acquired pneumonia in acute spinal cord injury

Respiratory complications, including pneumonia, are common during both acute care and initial rehabilitation after SCI. Their occurrence is closely associated with both acute care length of stay and hospitalization cost for

Table 3
Selected recommendations for prevention and management of hospital-acquired, ventilator-associated, and health care-associated pneumonia

Prevent person-to-person transmission of bacteria
- Use standard precautions, including hand washing, gloving for handling objects contaminated with respiratory secretions, and gowning when soiling with respiratory secretions is anticipated.
- Use aseptic technique and sterilized tubes when changing tracheostomy tubes.

Modify host risk factors for infection
- Administer pneumococcal vaccination to high-risk patients.
- Remove endotracheal, tracheal, and or/naso-enteric tubes as early as possible.
- Consider noninvasive positive-pressure ventilation in place of invasive ventilation.
- Perform orotracheal rather than nasotracheal intubation, unless contraindicated.
- Clear secretions above the endotracheal tube cuff before deflating the cuff.
- Unless contraindicated, elevate the head of the bed to 30 to 45 degrees for patients at high risk of aspiration who are receiving enteral tube feedings (note: this is typically contraindicated in patients with SCI because of risk of pressure ulcer formation secondary to skin shearing).

Prevent postoperative pneumonia
- Instruct preoperative high-risk patients on deep breathing exercises.
- Use incentive spirometry postoperatively.
- Remobilize patients out of bed as soon as medically feasible.

Diagnostic procedures
- Obtain chest radiographs to assist with confirming the diagnosis, assessing the severity, and ruling out associated complications such as pleural effusions.
- Obtain lower respiratory tract cultures.

Treatment
- Initiate appropriate broad-spectrum antibiotics as early as possible.
- Antibiotics should be chosen based on duration of hospitalization and the likelihood of multidrug-resistant antibiotics.
- Empiric antibiotics should include agents from a different antibiotic class than the patient has received recently.
- Consider narrowing the antibiotic coverage based on results of lower respiratory tract cultures and the patient's clinical response.
- For patients with uncomplicated pneumonia and a good clinical response to initially appropriate antibiotic therapy, consider a shorter treatment course (7 to 8 days) in the absence of nonfermenting gram-negative rods (eg, *Pseudomonas* or *Acinetobacter*).
- Perform serial assessments to monitor the clinical response. Patients who have not improved within 72 hours should be evaluated for noninfectious mimics of pneumonia, drug-resistant organisms, other sites of infection, and complications of pneumonia or its treatment, such as emphysema or *clostridium difficile* colitis.

Note: these recommendations are based on research performed in non-SCI patient populations. Except as noted, they are likely to apply to persons with acute or chronic SCI who have HAP or HCAP.

Data from American Thoracic Society and Infectious Disease Society of America. Guidelines for the management of adults with hospital-acquired, ventilator-associated, and health-care-associated pneumonia. Am J Respir Crit Care Med 2005;171(4):388–416 and Tablan O, Anderson L, Besser R, et al. Guidelines for preventing health-care–associated pneumonia, 2003: recommendations of CDC and the healthcare infection control practices advisory committee. MMWR Recomm Rep 2004;53(RR-3):1–36.

persons with new tetraplegia, and they are a more important determinant of cost than is the injury level [41]. Most published findings on pneumonia in persons with SCI come from patients undergoing acute care and initial rehabilitation at MSCIS hospitals. Jackson and Groomes [42] found a 31.4% rate of pneumonia during acute care and rehabilitation. Fishburn and colleagues [1] reported a combined rate of 50% for pneumonia or atelectasis during the first month after injury, with a 74% rate in patients with high-level tetraplegia. While receiving inpatient rehabilitation after acute care, 21.6% of patients with complete tetraplegia will have atelectasis or pneumonia [43]. Of note, 80% of pneumonias that develop soon after injury are left sided [1]. This has been attributed to difficulty with clearing secretions from the left bronchial tree using tracheal suctioning because of the more acute takeoff angle of the left mainstem bronchus.

There are no published data on etiologic organisms for pneumonia that develops during acute care or initial rehabilitation phases in person with SCI. These patients likely have a similar risk as other hospitalized patients for colonization with multidrug-resistant bacteria after 5 or more days of hospitalization. Therefore, the choice of empiric antibiotic coverage should be identical to that for HAP in neurologically intact patients and based in part on duration of hospitalization [23].

Hospital-acquired pneumonia in chronic spinal cord injury

The high incidence and case fatality for CAP is likely to be the primary reason that pneumonia is a leading cause of death after SCI. However, HAP could potentially account for a substantial proportion of the pneumonia-related deaths in persons with chronic SCI. To date, no studies have examined the epidemiology, pathogens, or risk factors for HAP in the chronically injured population. Many risk factors for HAP in the general population are prevalent in hospitalized persons with chronic SCI. These include expiratory dysfunction, prolonged antibiotic treatment, sedating medications, and supine position during feeding.

Summary

Respiratory infections are common in persons with SCI. Pneumonia, and to a lesser degree, acute bronchitis, are associated with significant morbidity and mortality. Guidelines for treatment of CAP were developed for use in the general population and may not be appropriate for persons with SCI. Optimal management of respiratory infections must take into account the severe expiratory dysfunction that is highly prevalent in this population as well as risk factors for HCAP in outpatients who have pneumonia. Persons with SCI should be informed of their risk of respiratory infections and be encouraged to seek prompt evaluation by physicians who are knowledgeable about complications of SCI.

References

[1] Fishburn M, Marino R, Ditunno JJ. Atelectasis and pneumonia in acute spinal cord injury. Arch Phys Med Rehabil 1990;71(3):197–200.

[2] DeVivo M, Krause J, Lammertse D. Recent trends in mortality and causes of death among persons with spinal cord injury. Arch Phys Med Rehabil 1999;80(11):1411–9.

[3] DeVivo M, Black K, Stover S. Causes of death during the first 12 years after spinal cord injury. Arch Phys Med Rehabil 1993;74(3):248–54.

[4] Minino A, Heron M, Smith B. Deaths: preliminary data for 2004. Natl Vital Stat Rep 2006; 54(19):1–49.

[5] Cardenas D, Hoffman J, Kirshblum S, et al. Etiology and incidence of rehospitalization after traumatic spinal cord injury: a multicenter analysis. Arch Phys Med Rehabil 2004;85(11): 1757–63.

[6] Dryden D, Saunders L, Rowe B, et al. Utilization of health services following spinal cord injury: a 6-year follow-up study. Spinal Cord 2004;42(9):513–25.

[7] Jackson A, Dijkers M, Devivo M, et al. A demographic profile of new traumatic spinal cord injuries: change and stability over 30 years. Arch Phys Med Rehabil 2004;85(11):1740–8.

[8] Smina M, Salam A, Khamiees M, et al. Cough peak flows and extubation outcomes. Chest 2003;124(1):262–8.

[9] Bach J, Saporito L. Criteria for extubation and tracheostomy tube removal for patients with ventilatory failure. A different approach to weaning. Chest 1996;110(6):1566–71.

[10] Agency for Healthcare Research and Quality. Treatment of pulmonary disease following cervical spinal cord injury. Rockville (MD): Agency for Healthcare Research and Quality; 2001.

[11] Schilero G, Grimm D, Bauman W, et al. Assessment of airway caliber and bronchodilator responsiveness in subjects with spinal cord injury. Chest 2005;127(1):149–55.

[12] Bhaskar K, Brown R, O'Sullivan D, et al. Bronchial mucus hypersecretion in acute quadriplegia. Macromolecular yields and glycoconjugate composition. Am Rev Respir Dis 1991; 143(3):640–8.

[13] Kirshblum S, Johnston M, Brown J, et al. Predictors of dysphagia after spinal cord injury. Arch Phys Med Rehabil 1999;80(9):1101–5.

[14] Neville A, Crookes P, Velmahos G, et al. Esophageal dysfunction in cervical spinal cord injury: a potentially important mechanism of aspiration. J Trauma 2005;59(4): 905–11.

[15] Campagnolo D, Bartlett J, Keller S. Influence of neurological level on immune function following spinal cord injury: a review. J Spinal Cord Med 2000;23(2):121–8.

[16] Trautner B, Atmar R, Hulstrom A, et al. Inactivated influenza vaccination for people with spinal cord injury. Arch Phys Med Rehabil 2004;85(11):1886–9.

[17] Darouiche R, Groover J, Rowland J, et al. Pneumococcal vaccination for patients with spinal cord injury. Arch Phys Med Rehabil 1993;74(12):1354–7.

[18] Laheij R, Sturkenboom M, Hassing R, et al. Risk of community-acquired pneumonia and use of gastric acid-suppressive drugs. JAMA 2004;292(16):1955–60.

[19] Bartlett J, Dowell S, Mandell L, et al. Practice guidelines for the management of community-acquired pneumonia in adults. Infectious Diseases Society of America. Clin Infect Dis 2000; 31(2):347–82.

[20] Garcia-Vazquez E, Marcos M, Mensa J, et al. Assessment of the usefulness of sputum culture for diagnosis of community-acquired pneumonia using the PORT predictive scoring system. Arch Intern Med 2004;164(16):1807–11.

[21] Centers for Disease Control and Prevention. Premature deaths, monthly mortality, and monthly physician contacts–United States. MMWR Morb Mortal Wkly Rep 1997;46(24): 556–61.

[22] Fine M, Auble T, Yealy D, et al. A prediction rule to identify low-risk patients with community-acquired pneumonia. N Engl J Med 1997;336(4):243–50.

[23] American Thoracic Society and Infectious Disease Society of America. Guidelines for the management of adults with hospital-acquired, ventilator-associated, and healthcare-associated pneumonia. Am J Respir Crit Care Med 2005;171(4):388–416.
[24] Smith B, Evans C, Kurichi J, et al. Acute respiratory infection visits in veterans with SCI&D: rates, trends and risk factors. J Spinal Cord Med, in press.
[25] Weaver F, Smith B, Evans C, et al. Outcomes of outpatient visits for acute respiratory illness in veterans with spinal cord injuries and disorders. Am J Phys Med Rehabil 2006;85(9): 718–26.
[26] Chang H, Evans C, Weaver F, et al. Etiology and outcomes of veterans with spinal cord injury and disorders hospitalized with community-acquired pneumonia. Arch Phys Med Rehabil 2005;86(2):262–7.
[27] Gilmore D, Bruce S, Jimenez E, et al. Pseudomonas aeruginosa colonization in patients with spinal cord injuries. J Clin Microbiol 1982;16(5):856–60.
[28] Arancibia F, Bauer T, Ewig S, et al. Community-acquired pneumonia due to gram-negative bacteria and pseudomonas aeruginosa: incidence, risk, and prognosis. Arch Intern Med 2002;162(16):1849–58.
[29] Rello J, Rue M, Jubert P, et al. Survival in patients with nosocomial pneumonia: impact of the severity of illness and the etiologic agent. Crit Care Med 1997;25(11):1862–7.
[30] Burns S, Weaver F, Parada J, et al. Management of community-acquired pneumonia in persons with spinal cord injury. Spinal Cord 2004;42(8):450–8.
[31] Glezen W, Greenberg S, Atmar R, et al. Impact of respiratory virus infections on persons with chronic underlying conditions. JAMA 2000;283(4):499–505.
[32] Falsey A, Hennessey P, Formica M, et al. Respiratory syncytial virus infection in elderly and high-risk adults. N Engl J Med 2005;352(17):1749–59.
[33] El-Sahly H, Atmar R, Glezen W, et al. Spectrum of clinical illness in hospitalized patients with "common cold" virus infections. Clin Infect Dis 2000;31(1):96–100.
[34] Bach J, Rajaraman R, Ballanger F, et al. Neuromuscular ventilatory insufficiency: effect of home mechanical ventilator use v oxygen therapy on pneumonia and hospitalization rates. Am J Phys Med Rehabil 1998;77(1):8–19.
[35] Gonzales R, Bartlett J, Besser R, et al. Principles of appropriate antibiotic use for treatment of uncomplicated acute bronchitis: background. Ann Emerg Med 2001;37(6):720–7.
[36] Advisory Committee on Immunization Practices. Prevention and control of influenza. MMWR Recomm Rep 2006;55(RR-10):1–42.
[37] Goldstein B, Weaver F, Hammond M. New CDC recommendations: annual influenza vaccination recommended for individuals with spinal cord injuries. J Spinal Cord Med 2005; 28(5):383–4.
[38] Advisory Committee on Immunization Practices. Prevention of pneumococcal disease. MMWR Recomm Rep 1997;46(RR-8):1–24.
[39] Jackson L, Neuzil K, Yu O, et al. Effectiveness of pneumococcal polysaccharide vaccine in older adults. N Engl J Med 2003;348(18):1747–55.
[40] Tablan O, Anderson L, Besser R, et al. Guidelines for preventing health-care–associated pneumonia, 2003: recommendations of CDC and the healthcare infection control practices advisory committee. MMWR Recomm Rep 2004;53(RR-3):1–36.
[41] Winslow C, Bode R, Felton D, et al. Impact of respiratory complications on length of stay and hospital costs in acute cervical spine injury. Chest 2002;121(5):1548–54.
[42] Jackson A, Groomes T. Incidence of respiratory complications following spinal cord injury. Arch Phys Med Rehabil 1994;75(3):270–5.
[43] Chen D, Apple DJ, Hudson L, et al. Medical complications during acute rehabilitation following spinal cord injury–current experience of the model systems. Arch Phys Med Rehabil 1999;80(11):1397–401.

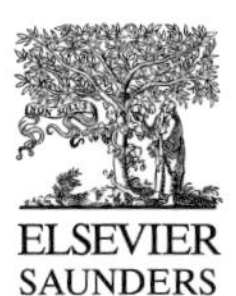
ELSEVIER
SAUNDERS

Phys Med Rehabil Clin N Am
18 (2007) 217–233

PHYSICAL MEDICINE AND REHABILITATION CLINICS OF NORTH AMERICA

Pain Following Spinal Cord Injury

Philip M. Ullrich, PhD

Veterans Affairs Puget Sound Healthcare System, SCI/D Services (128NAT), 1660 S. Columbian Way, Seattle, WA 98108, USA

Pain is common enough after spinal cord injury (SCI) to be considered an expected condition. Recent studies estimate the prevalence of pain after SCI to be between 77% and 81% [1–4]. Moreover, for many persons with SCI this pain is severe and has significant impact on daily functioning. Studies using standardized measures suggest that the intensity of pain is severe for between 20% and 33% of persons with pain after SCI [1,2]. Moderate to severe pain-related disability is found among 29% to 40% of persons with SCI who have pain [3,4]. The importance of pain to persons with SCI is further underscored by research that has consistently implicated pain in outcomes such as reduced quality of life, functional impairments, and depression [2,5–8]. Some studies have suggested that the impact of pain on quality of life (QOL) may be greater than that of the injury itself [9]. Pain conditions among persons with SCI tend to be stable over time, across studies with follow-up periods ranging from 2 to 10 years [2,3,10,11]. In fact, changes in a pain condition that do occur over time after SCI are likely to assume a worsening course [2,11].

Spinal cord injury pain types and taxonomies

SCI pain manifests in a multiplicity of forms; the typical patient experiences numerous types of pain that differ by location, qualitative descriptors, and purported etiology [4,7,8,12,13]. The complexity of SCI pain has direct bearing on its broad impact on functioning and resistance to treatment. Essential to clinical care of pain after SCI is the development of methods for

This work was supported by a grant from the Department of Veterans Affairs, Veterans Health Administration, Health Services Research and Development Service, Spinal Cord Injury Quality Enhancement Research Initiative (SCI QUERI, SCT 01-169).

This paper presents the views of the authors; it does not necessarily represent the views or policies of the Department of Veterans Affairs or the Health Services Research and Development Service.

E-mail address: philip.ullrich@va.gov

1047-9651/07/$ - see front matter
doi:10.1016/j.pmr.2007.03.001

rendering pain less mysterious and confusing, namely, valid and reliable methods for characterizing and categorizing pain. Development of valid and reliable SCI pain taxonomies has long been the aim of researchers. The sheer number of taxonomies that have been developed, and inconsistencies between taxonomies, underlines the complex and frustrating nature of pain after SCI. This section of the article will focus on common characteristics of the taxonomies and highlights a number of categorical systems that have been the subject of empirical studies of reliability.

Numerous pain types associated with spinal cord injury have been identified, primarily based on alleged causes, location of pain, and pain descriptors. Most taxonomic systems share two basic categories of pain after SCI: musculoskeletal/nociceptive and neuropathic/neurologic. As a major category, neuropathic pain is prevalent in 30% to 40% of persons with SCI five or more years after injury [3,14]. Musculoskeletal pain appears to be more common, occurring in 50% to 60% of persons with SCI five or more years after injury [3,14]. However, when "worst" SCI pains are identified, the majority (50% to 56%) are likely to be neuropathic, as opposed to musculoskeletal [14]. SCI pain types and subtypes are presented in Table 1 [15,16] according to the major classification systems.

Musculoskeletal pain refers to pain originating from damage to tissue and bone structures and may include the following pain subtypes. In the immediate aftermath of injury the sources of pain may be obviously related to bone, joint, and tissue trauma. Also, pain may stem from fractured vertebrae and torn ligaments that destabilize the spine. Pain related to spine instability is affected by positioning and activity. Muscle spasm pain may arise long after the injury. Overuse pain, or pressure syndromes, typically occur in areas of normal sensation and high activity, such as the shoulder.

Neuropathic pain (also called neurologic or central pain) is directly attributable to spinal cord damage and has been divided further into a number of subtypes. One subtype of neuropathic pain, SCI pain, is typically perceived below the level of injury in areas without normal sensation. Transition zone pain occurs at the level of injury and may include pain caused by nerve entrapment. Radicular pain is neuropathic pain occurring at the level of injury caused by nerve root damage related to the initial injury or subsequent irritation. Visceral pain occurs in the abdominal region, typically well after initial injury and often in the absence of visceral pathology. Visceral pain is considered neurologic/neuropathic in some classification systems. However, causes of visceral pain can include conditions such as bowel and urinary tract obstruction, renal calculi, or other intra-abdominal pathologies, suggesting that visceral pain may be categorized better as nociceptive pain in some cases.

Reliability of spinal cord injury pain classification schemes

Although there are numerous ways to determine a classification system's reliability, most studies have focused on interrater reliability, meaning the

Table 1
SCI pain types according to major classification schemes

Bryce/Ragnarsson [20]	Cardenas [14]	Donovan [15]	IASP [22]	Tunks [16]
Above level	Neurologic	(1) Segmental	Nociceptive	Above level
(1) Nociceptive	(1) Spinal cord	(2) Spinal cord	(1) Musculoskeletal	(1) Myofascial
(2) Neuropathic	(2) Transition zone	(3) Visceral	(2) Visceral	(2) Syringomyelia
At level	(3) Radicular	(4) Mechanical	Neuropathic	(3) Non–spinal cord injury
(3) Nociceptive	(4) Visceral	(5) Psychogenic	(3) Above level	At level
(4) Neuropathic	Musculoskeletal		(4) At level	(4) Radicular
Below level	(5) Mechanical spine		(5) Below level	(5) Hyperalgesic border reaction
(5) Nociceptive	(6) Overuse			(6) Fracture
(6) Neuropathic				(7) Myofascial (incomplete)
				Below level
				(8) Diffuse burning
				(9) Phantom
				(10) Visceral
				(11) Myofascial (incomplete)

degree of agreement between two raters of the same variable. Reliability of a pain classification system is fundamental for determining the system's validity, meaning the degree to which the system is measuring what it purports to measure. Interrater reliability is commonly indexed as a Kappa coefficient, having a range from −1.0 to 1.0, with 1.0 indicating perfect agreement between raters. Values greater than .60 [17] or .70 [18] are considered to represent adequate interrater reliability. As seen in Table 2, the interrater reliability of major SCI pain classification systems has been modest, at best, across independent studies. Across classification systems, raters disagree on the classification of between 20% and 50% of pain sites. The apparent differences in performance of these classification systems may be caused by variability in the complexity of systems in terms of how many pain types and subtypes are included. As noted by Putzke and colleagues [19], the reliability of classification systems increases as the number of pain types decreases. Classification systems show better interrater reliability when broad pain types are considered, such as nociceptive-neuropathic [19] or location of pain relative to injury level [20]. Also, it is important to note that methodologic differences between studies in Table 2 may have bearing on results. Specifically, interrater reliability for the Bryce and colleagues [20] system reflected comparisons between physicians recruited for the study and the investigators themselves. In the study of the Cardenas [14] system, interrater reliability was based on ratings of questionnaire data. However, in a subset of ratings made using information gained from clinical interview and physical examination, the Kappa coefficient was comparable though somewhat reduced (.66 compared with .68 with questionnaire data).

Use of verbal descriptors to categorize pain may also have bearing on the limited reliability of classification systems. Verbal pain descriptors, while being a standard method for classifying SCI pain, actually have limited utility in discriminating between pain types. A number of investigators [14,21] have found considerable overlap in verbal descriptors for broad pain types. For example, each verbal descriptor (eg, burning, aching, shooting, stabbing, tingling) may be endorsed at least 8% of the time for each of the most common pain types across classification systems [21]. Cardenas and colleagues

Table 2
Reliability of SCI pain classification systems

	Kappa coefficient	Percent agreement
Bryce and colleagues [20]	.70	Unavailable
Cardenas [14]	.68	Unavailable
Donovan [15]	.55	50%–62%
IASP [22]	.49	52%
Tunks [16]	.49	27%

Kappa coefficient is the proportion of agreement controlling for chance agreement, with 1.0 representing perfect agreement between raters. Kappa coefficients greater than .60 or .70 reflect substantial interrater agreement.

[14] found that "aching", a term typically thought to be descriptive of musculoskeletal pain generally and overuse pain specifically, was also used by patients to describe 64% to 67% of pains classified as neuropathic during examination.

Various SCI pain classification systems may be adequate for identifying the two broad types of pain, musculoskeletal and neuropathic, but additional research is required to develop more reliable taxonomic methods.

Psychological aspects of spinal cord injury pain

Absent from most classification systems is the concept of a pain type that is purely psychological in origin. Rather, psychological factors such as mood, thoughts, and social interactions may be considered to have a bidirectional relationship with all types of pain, with particularly important roles in the development of chronic pain and pain-related functional disability [22]. As noted earlier in this chapter, most if not all persons with SCI endure pain on a daily basis for years, and yet only a minority experience clinically meaningful pain-related functional disability. Understanding the differential impact of pain on functioning across individuals is an important goal for research, with direct bearing on allocation of health care resources and the design of more effective interventions. With this aim in mind, numerous investigators have examined what demographic, medical, or SCI-related factors might predict variability in the functional impact of pain. Consistent predictors of pain-related disability have not emerged from these studies, as noted in past reviews that span decades of research [23,24]. One explanation for the inconsistent findings relates to methodologic problems across studies, such as small sample sizes, cross-sectional designs, and variability in how pain-related disability is defined and measured. Alternatively, consistent findings may be elusive if variability in pain-related disability is largely accounted for by psychological factors. For example, a well-replicated finding in both cross-sectional and longitudinal studies is that psychological factors, such as mood or cognitions, are better predictors of pain interference than injury-related factors such as level, completeness, or etiology of injury [25–27].

These findings have stimulated research and theorizing regarding explanatory models of psychological factors and pain-related disability. Prominent in this research have been theories emphasizing the role of maladaptive cognitive processes, such as catastrophizing, in the development and maintenance of functional disability related to pain. Catastrophizing refers to exaggerated negative expectations or interpretations of an experience, such as pain [28]. The degree to which one catastrophizes ("I cannot stand this pain! It will never get better!") is thought to be associated with the impact of pain on outcomes such as functioning and well-being. Strong associations between catastrophizing and functioning have been observed across diverse patient groups while controlling for possible confounds

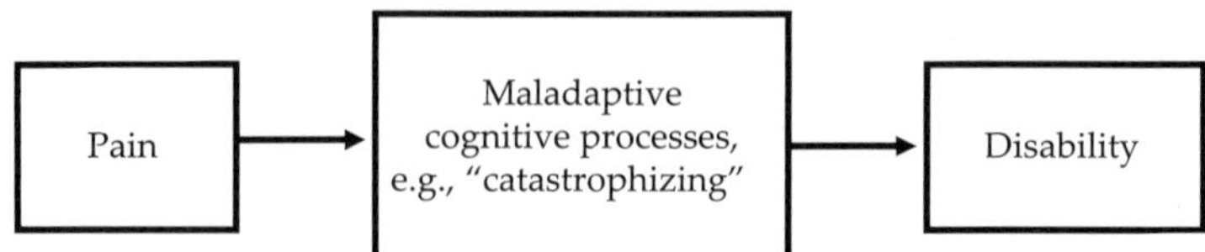

Fig. 1. Associations between pain, cognitions, and pain-related disability.

such as pain severity, illness severity, or personality [28]. Consistent with research among other populations, catastrophizing has been shown to be a potent predictor of pain-related functional disability among persons with SCI [27]. Catastrophizing is thought to play a mediating role between pain and functioning in most models. For example, painful stimuli may serve to activate "pain schemas," or memory stores of knowledge related to pain, that support cognitive-processing biases such as catastrophizing [29]. Biases in cognitive processing may involve enhanced memory for, or attention toward, negatively valenced illness-related information [29]. The effect of cognitive processing biases such as catastrophizing may be to heighten the threat value of pain and highlight inadequacies in personal coping resources, with ultimate impact on activity levels and function (Fig. 1; [28,29]).

The impact of pain on psychological adjustment is also important to describe. Cross-sectional, correlational studies consistently show associations between pain and various indicators of psychosocial adjustment after SCI [2,5–8]. While this evidence supports causal hypotheses regarding the effect of pain on psychosocial adjustment of persons with SCI, it may be just as likely that psychosocial adjustment is influencing pain. However, prospective studies suggest that pain may precede conditions reflective of psychosocial maladjustment, such as clinical depression [30].

Assessment of spinal cord injury pain

Medical assessment

Pain assessment procedures that have been detailed elsewhere [31–33] are reviewed here. Assessment of pain in persons with SCI should begin with classification of the pain according to mechanism to suggest the most appropriate first-line treatment strategies. Most classification systems rely on neurologic level determined by examination and verbal descriptions of pain locations (eg, above, at, or below level) and pain qualities (eg, burning, aching, stabbing). Thus, neurologic examination and a detailed pain interview are arguably the central aspects of SCI pain assessment. However, medical examination should also include general physical, musculoskeletal, laboratory (radiologic, electrophysiologic) and mental status testing. Information should be gathered regarding a patient's family, psychosocial, and medical histories. A pain history should be taken to understand the characteristics of the pain at onset, circumstances surrounding onset, past treatments, and the course of pain to the present date. The interview should elicit a detailed pain description by the patient, in terms of pain location, distribution, quality, intensity, periodicity, and duration. Factors aggravating or relieving pain should be noted, eg, movement, pressure, heat-cold, or stress. Pain description is accompanied by physical examination of the pain through inspection and palpation of the painful region. Physical examination should also assess for allodynia, hyperalgesia, or hyperesthesia in painful regions using appropriate brush, pinch, pin-prick, or scratch tests. A physical therapist is ideally involved in SCI pain assessment to determine biomechanical origins of pain, such as gait, postural, or seating abnormalities.

Self-report measures

Pain assessment should always include reliable and valid self-report measures that reflect the biopsychosocial nature of pain. Self-report measures compliment information derived from interview and supply essential data for evaluating the course of pain over time and response to treatment. The numerical rating scale (NRS; 0-10) of pain intensity is by far the most commonly used measure of pain. A number of studies have established the NRS as a reliable [34] and valid [35,36] measure of pain intensity. Moreover, NRS pain intensity scores may be classified into mild, moderate, and severe categories [35]. Beyond pain intensity it is important for assessment to capture the multidimensional nature of pain in terms of interference with daily activities. Specifically, the Initiative on Methods, Measurement, and Pain Assessment in Clinical Trials group (IMMPACT; [37]) recommended that measures of pain severity, physical functioning, and emotional functioning be included in all clinical trials of chronic pain interventions. The impact of pain on physical functioning may be captured by pain interference measures: the Graded Chronic Pain Disability scale [38], the Brief Pain Inventory [39], and the Multidimensional Pain Inventory (MPI; [40]) have all shown adequate reliability and validity in SCI populations [41–43]. The impact of pain on emotional functioning may be assessed by a measure of depressive symptoms such as the Beck Depression Inventory (BDI; [44]) or a broader measure of mood disturbance such as the Profile of Mood states [45]. The Patient Health Questionnaire [46] may be an especially useful tool, because it produces a score reflecting depression symptom severity based on questions matching the nine diagnostic criteria that make up the Diagnostic and Statistical Manual of Mental Disorders, 4th Edition (DSM-IV; [47]) criteria for major depression. Furthermore, the Patient Health Questionnaire (PHQ-9) has support for its validity in the SCI population [48].

Psychological assessment

Self-report measures of pain experiences should be accompanied by a clinical interview and additional testing that systematically evaluates psychological concomitants of pain. An interview should address mental health history, substance use/misuse history, and aspects of psychosocial history not previously pursued by other team members. Similarly, current mental health concerns and treatments, psychiatric diagnoses, drug and alcohol use patterns, and psychosocial stressors should all be appraised. The Minnesota Multiphasic Personality Inventory (MMPI; [49]) has been used for standardized assessment of longstanding patterns of affect, thought, and behavior among persons with SCI [50,51]. Neuropsychological testing may be indicated to explore questions of cognitive functioning, particularly in the presence of high injury levels or other risk factors for brain injury.

Treatment of spinal cord injury pain

As noted earlier in this chapter, SCI pain tends to assume a stable or even worsening course over the years following initial injury. Importantly, the generally unfavorable trajectory for SCI pain occurs in spite of the fact that in most cases pain is being actively treated. Therefore, it is not surprising that patient satisfaction with pain treatments is low [52–55]. A review of controlled clinical trials for SCI pain may help explain the results of patient satisfaction studies. Controlled trials of pain treatments among people with SCI are surprisingly rare given the high prevalence and impact of pain in this population [56]. Those controlled trials that have been published tend to have small sample sizes and other methodologic flaws, perhaps accounting for the fact that it is not surprising that many have failed to reject the null hypothesis. As seen in Table 3 [57–71], only 12 of 22 (55%) treatments tested in controlled clinical trials have shown benefits over placebo. In 2001, McMaster University's Evidence-based Practice Center prepared an evidence report on the management of neuropathic pain after SCI, concluding that (1) the reliability and validity of SCI pain measurement strategies are unknown, and (2) poor methods used in the few studies of SCI pain treatments that have been conducted preclude proper evaluation of treatment effects [72].

Since the publication of the McMaster's report, the number of published, controlled clinical trials for SCI pain treatments has nearly doubled (see Table 3), and numerous psychometric investigations of SCI pain classification systems have been conducted [19,20,73,74]. Although the increased volume and quality of this research is encouraging, the situation for the practicing clinician remains essentially the same as it was a decade ago: there are no proven reliable and valid standards for assessing and categorizing SCI pain, nor are there routinely effective treatments for SCI pain. Because of these issues, case reports, uncontrolled trials, and research from other conditions often are considered as part of the evidence base for selecting SCI pain treatments [75,76].

Reviews and algorithms of SCI pain treatments [76–78] share two common features: (1) an emphasis that the effectiveness of treatment is dependent on identification of the correct types of pain and (2) recommendations that treatments be multimodal and interdisciplinary. First-line treatments for SCI pain will be considered here briefly; more detailed reviews can be found in the publications cited earlier.

Musculoskeletal pain

Pain related to spine instability may be alleviated by immobilization and surgery (eg, spinal fusion) to correct the instability. Musculoskeletal pain can also be caused by posture, seating, or gait abnormalities that may be correctable through retraining and equipment modification. Overuse pain may be addressed by physical therapy [79], nonsteroidal anti-inflammatory drugs (NSAIDs), or opioids. Muscle spasms are a frequent source of pain after SCI, indicating the need for oral or intrathecal antispasticity medications such as baclofen.

Visceral pain

Visceral pain may be attributable to bowel or bladder dysfunction such as urinary tract infection, bowel impaction, or obstructions in the urinary system, with treatments being aimed to eliminate the source.

Neuropathic pain

First-line treatments for neuropathic pain are anticonvulsants such as gabapentin, carbamazepine, or pregabalin. Tricyclic antidepressants (TCAs), such as amitriptyline or nortriptyline, have been prescribed commonly for neuropathic pain after SCI. Evidence for the efficacy of TCAs for neuropathic pain comes from non-SCI populations; one trial among SCI patients found no benefit from the TCA amitriptyline [80]. Siddall and Middleton [76] suggest that TCAs combined with anticonvulsants may be more effective than either drug class administered alone. Opioid medications such as oxycodone and methadone are commonly used for both acute and chronic neuropathic pain.

Surgical treatments

Surgical treatments such as spine fusion or nerve decompression are useful in treating SCI pain originating in spine instability or syringomyelia, respectively. Ablative procedures such as cordotomy, cordectomy, and myelotomy are recognized generally as being controversial, at best. Uncontrolled case reports have shown that these procedures may have limited utility in controlling pain after SCI and furthermore may aggravate pain and other conditions such as bladder dysfunction or spasticity. Another ablative procedure, dorsal root entry zone lesion (DREZ), is thought to be indicated for some cases of neuropathic pain at the level of injury.

Table 3
Controlled trials of different treatments for SCI pain

Trial	Pain type	Treatment	Design, N	Outcome	NNT
Anticonvulsants					
Drewes, et al, 1994 [57]	Neur	Valproate, 600–2400 mg	Cross-over[a], 20	Valproate = placebo	ns
Finnerup, et al, 2002 [58]	Neur	Lamotrigine, 200–400 mg	Cross-over, 22	Lamotrigine = placebo	ns
Levendoglu, et al, 2004 [59]	Neur	Gabapentin, 1900–3600 mg	Cross-over, 20	Gabapentin > placebo	NA
Siddall, et al, 2006 [60]	Neur	Pregabalin, 150–600 mg	Parallel, 70	Pregabalin > placebo	7.1
Antidepressants					
Cardenas, et al, 2002 [80]	Mixed	Amitryptyline, 50 mg	Parallel, 84	Amitryptyline = placebo	ns
Davidoff, et al, 1987 [61]	Neur	Trazadone, 150 mg	Parallel, 18	Trazadone = placebo	ns
Cranial electrotherapy stimulation (CES)					
Capel, et al, 2003 [81]	Mixed	12 μA, 4 hours/day, 4 days	Crossover, 27	CES > placebo	NA
Fregni, et al, 2006 [82]	Mixed	2 mA, 20 min/day, 5 days	Parallel, 17	CES > placebo	2.1
Tan, et al, 2006 [83]	Mixed	100 μA, 1 hour/day, 21 days	Parallel, 38	CES > placebo	NA
Exercise					
Curtis, et al, 1999 [79]	Shoulder	6 months daily sessions	Parallel, 42	Exer > placebo	NA
Martin-Ginis, et al, 2003 [62]	Mixed	24 twice-weekly sessions	Parallel, 34	Exer > placebo	NA
GABA-A agonists					
Canavero & Bonicalzi, 2004 [63]	SCI & Stroke	Propofol, i.v., 0.2 mg/kg	Cross-over[a], 21	Propofol > placebo	2.0

NMDA-receptor antagonists					
Eide, et al, 1995 [64]	Neur	Ketamine, i.v., 180 μg,	Cross-over, 9	Ketamine > placebo	NA
Eide, et al, 1995 [64]	Neur	Alfentanil, i.v., 19 μg,	Cross-over, 9	Alfentanil > placebo	NA
Kvarnstrom, et al, 2004 [65]	Neur	Ketamine, i.v., .4 mg/kg	Crossover, 10	Ketamine > placebo	2.0
Opioids					
Attal, et al, 2002 [66]	SCI & Stroke	Morphine, i.v., 16 mg	Cross-over, 9	Morphine = placebo	3.0
Siddall, et al, 2000 [67]	Neur	Morphine, i.t., .75 mg,	Cross-over, 15	Morphine = placebo	ns
Siddall, et al, 2000 [67]	Neur	Clonidine, i.t., 50 μg,	Cross-over, 15	Clonidine = Placebo	ns
Siddall, et al, 2000 [67]	Neur	Morphine, i.t., .75 mg and Clonidine, i.t., 50 μg,	Cross-over, 15	Morphine/Clonidine > placebo	7.5
Sodium channel blockers/local analgesic					
Attal, et al, 2000 [68]	SCI & Stroke	Lidocaine, i.v., 5 mg/kg	Cross-over, 10	Lidocaine > placebo	5.0
Chiou-Tan, et al, 1996 [69]	Neur	Mexiletine, 450 mg	Cross-over, 11	Mexiletine = placebo	NA
Finnerup, et al, 2005 [70]	Neur	Lidocaine, 5 mg/kg	Cross-over, 24	Lidocaine > placebo	3.0
Kvarnstrom, et al, 2004 [65]	Neur	Lidocaine, 2.5 mg/kg	Cross-over, 10	Lidocaine > placebo	10.0
Loubser, et al, 1996 [71]	Neur	Lidocaine, 50–100 mg	Cross-over, 21	Lidocaine > placebo	3.5

Abbreviations: exer, exercise; i.v., intravenous; i.t., intrathecal; Mixed, neuropathic and musculoskeletal; NA, data not available from the report; Neur, neuropathic; NNT, number needed to treat to provide one patient with at least 50% pain relief; ns, non-significant.

[a] Nonrandomized design.

Electrical stimulation

Transcutaneous electrical nerve stimulation (TENS) or spinal cord stimulation may offer some relief of pain at the level of injury in areas with partial sensation. Electrical stimulation of the brain has long been considered an option of last resort [24], but recent years have seen three randomized, controlled clinical trials of cranial electrotherapy stimulation with positive impact on pain after SCI [81–83].

Psychological treatments

Major reviews [76–78] of treatments for SCI pain recognize that psychological factors have direct effects on the experience and consequences of pain and therefore recommend that psychological treatments be considered an option for managing all types of pain after SCI. As is the case for physical/pharmacologic therapies, the evidence base informing selection of psychological treatments for pain after SCI is largely based on case reports, uncontrolled studies, and studies among non-SCI populations. Meta-analysis of randomized, controlled trials conducted in the general population shows that the effects of cognitive-behavioral therapy on chronic pain are comparable in magnitude to pharmacologic intervention [84]. No randomized, clinical trials of psychological treatments for pain in persons with SCI have been published to date. However, positive reports have come from pain treatment pilot projects emphasizing cognitive-behavioral principles [85–87] and a case series of hypnotic analgesia treatments for pain in SCI [88]. Other trials of psychological treatments for pain in persons with SCI are underway (cf., [56,89,90]).

Patients' attitudes may have bearing on implementation of psychological treatments in real-world settings. Findings suggest that persons with SCI view psychological treatments as having effects on pain problems that are weak relative to other treatments [53,55]. Furthermore, medical patients [91] including those with SCI [92,93], may be generally disinterested in psychological problems or interventions. However, when patients with SCI have been queried directly regarding their interest in psychological or nonpharmacologic treatments for pain, they have expressed greater interest in psychological treatments than other options such as opioids [89,90].

Interdisciplinary care

Interdisciplinary intervention is frequently postulated to be the best approach to treating SCI pain in major reviews [76–78]. In fact, the Rehabilitation Accreditation Commission [94] specifies that an interdisciplinary approach is preferred in all aspects of rehabilitation care. In non-SCI populations, interdisciplinary treatments have proven to be superior to single-discipline care [95]. Gironda [86] reported on a pilot project of an interdisciplinary intervention for shoulder pain among persons with SCI. The interdisciplinary program focused on functional preservation through medical, physical therapy, recreational therapy, and cognitive behavioral psychotherapy components. This report is novel and important for its detailed summary of interdisciplinary care for SCI pain as well as the focus on shoulder pain.

Summary

Pain is one of the most common complications after SCI and is notoriously difficult to assess and treat. Effective treatment strategies must build from systematic assessment and categorization of pain in spite of the limitations to current classification systems. A number of pain measures with strong psychometric properties are now available to assist in characterizing pain and its comorbidities to provide better monitoring of intervention effects. The number and quality of controlled trials of interventions for SCI pain is increasing and broadening beyond investigations of pharmaceutical treatments.

References

[1] Finnerup NB, Johannesen IL, Sindrup SH, et al. Pain and dysesthesia in patients with spinal cord injury: a postal survey. Spinal Cord 2001;39(5):256–62.

[2] Jensen MP, Hoffman AJ, Cardenas DD. Chronic pain in persons with spinal cord injury: a survey and longitudinal study. Spinal Cord 2005;43(12):704–12.

[3] Siddall PJ, McClelland JM, Rutkowski SB, et al. A longitudinal study of the prevalence and characteristics of pain in the first 5 years following spinal cord injury. Pain 2003;103(3): 249–57.

[4] Turner JA, Cardenas DD, Warms CA, et al. Chronic pain associated with spinal cord injuries: a community survey. Arch Phys Med Rehabil 2001;82(4):501–9.

[5] Cairns DM, Adkins RH, Scott MD. Pain and depression in acute traumatic spinal cord injury: origins of chronic problematic pain? Arch Phys Med Rehabil 1996;77:329–35.

[6] Rintala DH, Loubser PG, Castro J, et al. Chronic pain in a community-based sample of men with spinal cord injury: prevalence, severity, and relationship with impairment, disability, handicap, and subjective well-being. Arch Phys Med Rehabil 1998;79:604–14.

[7] Turner JA, Cardenas DD. Chronic pain problems in individuals with spinal cord injuries. Semin Clin Neuropsychiatry 1999;4(3):186–94.

[8] Widerstrom-Noga EG, Felipe-Cuervo E, Yezierski RP. Chronic pain after spinal injury: interference with sleep and daily activities. Arch Phys Med Rehabil 2001;82(11):1571–7.

[9] Westgren N, Levi R. Quality of life and traumatic spinal cord injury. Arch Phys Med Rehabil 1998;79:1433–9.

[10] Cruz-Almeida Y, Martinez-Arizala A, Widerstrom-Noga EG. Chronicity of pain associated with spinal cord injury: a longitudinal analysis. J Rehabil Res Dev 2005;42(5):585–94.

[11] Rintala DH, Hart KA, Priebe MM. Predicting consistency of pain over a 10-year period in persons with spinal cord injury. J Rehabil Res Dev 2004;41(1):75–88.

[12] Siddall PJ, Taylor DA, McClelland JM, et al. Pain report and the relationship of pain to physical factors in the first 6 months following spinal cord injury. Pain 1999;81(1–2):187–97.

[13] Stormer S, Gerner HJ, Gruninger W, et al. Chronic pain/dysaesthesiae in spinal cord injury patients: results of a multicentre study. Spinal Cord 1997;35(7):446–55.

[14] Cardenas DD, Turner JA, Warms CA, et al. Classification of chronic pain associated with spinal cord injuries. Arch Phys Med Rehabil 2002;83:1708–14.
[15] Donovan WH, Dimitrijevic MR, Dahm L, et al. Neurophysiological approaches to chronic pain following spinal cord injury. Paraplegia 1982;20:135–46.
[16] Tunks E. Pain in spinal cord injured patients. In: Bloch RF, Basbaum M, editors. Management of spinal cord injuries. Baltimore (MD): Williams and Wilkins; 1986. p. 180–211.
[17] Landis JR, Koch GG. The measurement of observer agreement for categorical data. Biometrics 1977;33:159–74.
[18] Cramer D. Fundamental statistics for social research. New York, Routledge; 1998.
[19] Putzke JD, Richards JS, Ness T, et al. Interrater reliability of the International Association for the Study of Pain and Tunk's spinal cord injury pain classification schemes. Am J Phys Med Rehabil 2003;82(6):437–40.
[20] Bryce TN, Dijkers MP, Ragnarsson KT, et al. Reliability of the Bryce/Ragnarsson spinal cord injury pain taxonomy. J Spinal Cord Med 2006;29(2):118–32.
[21] Putzke JD, Richards JS, Hicken BL, et al. Pain classification following spinal cord injury: the utility of verbal descriptors. Spinal Cord 2002;40:118–27.
[22] Siddall PJ, Yezierski RP, Loeser JD. Taxonomy and epidemiology of spinal cord injury pain. In: Yezierski RP, Burchiel KJ, editors. Spinal cord injury pain: assessment, mechanisms, management. Seattle (WA): IASP Press; 2002. p. 9–24.
[23] Mariano AJ. Chronic pain and spinal cord injury. Clin J Pain 1992;8:87–92.
[24] Siddall PJ, Loeser J. Pain following spinal cord injury. Spinal Cord 2001;39:63–73.
[25] Putzke JD, Richards JS, Hicken BL, et al. Interference due to pain following spinal cord injury: important predictors and impact on quality of life. Pain 2002;100:231–42.
[26] Richards JS, Meredith RL, Nepomuceno C, et al. Psycho-social aspects of chronic pain in spinal cord injury. Pain 1980;8(3):355–66.
[27] Turner JA, Jensen MP, Warms CA, et al. Catastrophizing is associated with pain intensity, psychological distress, and pain-related disability among individuals with chronic pain after spinal cord injury. Pain 2002;98(1):127–34.
[28] Sullivan MJ, Thorn B, Haythornthwaite JA, et al. Theoretical perspectives on the relation between catastrophizing and pain. Clin J Pain 2001;17:52–64.
[29] Pincus T, Morley S. Cognitive-processing bias in chronic pain: a review and integration Psychol Bull 2001;127(5):599–617.
[30] Banks SM, Kerns RD. Explaining high rates of depression in chronic pain: a diathesis-stress framework. Psychol Bull 1996;119(1):95–110.
[31] Loeser JD, Butler SH, Chapman CR, et al. Bonica's management of pain. 3rd edition. Seattle (WA): Lippincott Williams & Wilkins; 2001.
[32] Wegener ST, Elliott TR. Pain assessment in spinal cord injury. Clin J Pain 1992;8: 93–101.
[33] Widerstrom-Noga EG. Evaluation of clinical characteristics of pain and psychosocial factors after spinal cord injury. In: Yezierski RP, Burchiel KJ, editors. Spinal cord injury pain: assessment, mechanisms, management. Seattle (WA): IASP Press; 2002. p. 53–82.
[34] Jensen MP, Turner JA, Romano JM. Fisher LD. Comparative reliability and validity of chronic pain intensity measures. Pain 1999;83(2):157–62.
[35] Hanley MA, Masedo A, Jensen MP, et al. Pain interference in persons with spinal cord injury: classification of mild, moderate, and severe pain. J Pain 2006;7(2):129–33.
[36] Hanley MA, Jensen MP, Ehde DM, et al. Clinically significant change in pain intensity ratings in persons with spinal cord injury or amputation. Clin J Pain 2006;22(1):25–31.
[37] Turk DC, Dworkin RH, Allen RR, et al. Core outcome domains for chronic pain clinical trials: IMMPACT recommendations. Pain 2003;106:337–45.
[38] Von Korff M, Ormel J, Keefe FJ, et al. Grading the severity of chronic pain. Pain 1992;50: 133–49.
[39] Cleeland CS, Ryan KM. Pain assessment: global use of the Brief Pain Inventory. Ann Acad Med 1994;23:129–38.

[40] Kerns RD, Turk DC, Rudy TE. The West Haven-Yale Multidimensional Pain Inventory (WHYMPI). Pain 1985;23:345–56.
[41] Raichle KA, Osborne TL, Jensen MP, et al. The reliability and validity of pain interference measures in persons with spinal cord injury. J Pain 2006;17(3):179–86.
[42] Widerstrom-Noga EG, Duncan R, Felipe-Cruz E, et al. Assessment of the impact of pain and impairments associated with spinal cord injuries. Arch Phys Med Rehabil 2002;83: 395–404.
[43] Widerstrom-Noga EG, Cruz-Almeida Y, Martinez-Arizala A, et al. Internal consistency, stability, and validity of the spinal cord injury version of the Multidimensional Pain Inventory. Arch Phys Med Rehabil 2006;87:516–23.
[44] Beck AT, Ward CH, Mendelson M, et al. An inventory for measuring depression. Arch Gen Psychiatry 1961;4:561–71.
[45] McNair DM, Lorr M, Droppleman LF. Profile of mood states. San Diego (CA): Educational and Industrial Testing Service; 1971.
[46] Kroenke K, Spitzer RL, Williams JB. The PHQ-9 validity of a brief depression symptom severity measure. J Gen Intern Med 2001;16:606–13.
[47] American Psychiatric Association. Diagnostic and statistical manual of mental disorders. 4th edition. Washington, DC: APA; 1994.
[48] Bombardier CH, Richards JS, Krause JS, et al. Symptoms of major depression in people with spinal cord injury: implications for screening. Arch Phys Med Rehabil 2004;85(11):1749–56.
[49] Butcher JN, Dahlstrom WG, Graham JR, et al. MMPI-2(Minnesota Multiphasic Personality Inventory-2): manual for administration and scoring. Minneapolis (MN): University of Minnesota Press; 1989.
[50] Barncord SW, Wanlass RL. A correction procedure for the Minnesota Multiphasic Personality Inventory-2 for persons with spinal cord injury. Arch Phys Med Rehabil 2000;81(9): 1185–90.
[51] Kendall PC, Edinger J, Eberly C. Taylor's MMPI correction factor for spinal cord injury: empirical endorsement. J Consult Clin Psychol 1978;35:183–8.
[52] Cardenas DD, Jensen MP. Treatments for chronic pain in persons with spinal cord injury: a survey study. J Spinal Cord Med. 2006;29(2):109–17.
[53] Warms CA, Turner JA, Marshall HM, et al. Treatments for chronic pain associated with spinal cord injuries: many are tried, few are helpful. Clin J Pain 2002;18(3):154–63.
[54] Murphy D, Reid DB. Pain treatment satisfaction in spinal cord injury. Spinal Cord 2001;39: 44–6.
[55] Widerstrom-Noga EG, Turk DC. Types and effectiveness of treatments used by people with chronic pain associated with spinal cord injuries: influence of pain and psychosocial characteristics. Spinal Cord 2003;41(11):600–9.
[56] Richards JS. Spinal cord injury pain: impact, classification, treatment trends, and implications from translational research. Rehabil Psychol 2005;50(2):99–102.
[57] Drewes AM, Andreasen A, Poulsen LH. Valproate for treatment of chronic central pain after spinal cord injury: a double-blind cross-over study. Paraplegia 1994;32:565–9.
[58] Finnerup NB, Sindrup SH, Bach FW, et al. Lamotrigine in spinal cord injury pain: a randomized controlled trial. Pain 2002;96:375–83.
[59] Levendoglu F, Ogun CO, Ozerbil O, et al. Gabapentin is a first line drug for the treatment of neuropathic pain in spinal cord injury. Spine 2004;29:743–51.
[60] Siddall PJ, Cousins MD, Otte A, et al. Pregabalin in central neuropathic pain associated with spinal cord injury: a placebo-controlled trial. Neurology 2006;67:1792–800.
[61] Davidoff G, Guarracini M, Roth E, et al. Trazadone hydrochloride in the treatment of dysesthetic pain in traumatic myelopathy: a randomized, double-blind, placebo-controlled study. Pain 1987;29:151–61.
[62] Martin-Ginis KA, Latimer AE, McKechnie K, et al. Using exercise to enhance subjective well-being among people with spinal cord injury: the mediating influences of stress and pain. Rehabil Psychol 2003;48(3):157–64.

[63] Canavero S, Bonicalzi V. Intravenous subhypnotic propofol in central pain: a double-blind, placebo-controlled, crossover study. Clin Neuropharmacol. 2004;27(4):182–6.
[64] Eide PK, Stubhaug A, Stenehjem AE. Central dysesthesia pain after traumatic spinal cord injury is dependent on N-methyl-D-aspartate receptor activation. Neurosurgery 1995; 37(6):1080–7.
[65] Kvarnstrom A, Karlsten R, Quiding H, et al. The analgesic effect of intravenous ketamine and lidocaine on pain after spinal cord injury. Acta Anaesthesiol Scand 2004;48(4): 498–506.
[66] Attal N, Guirimand F, Brasseur L, et al. Effects of IV morphine in central pain: a randomized placebo-controlled study. Neurology 2002;58(4):554–63.
[67] Siddall PJ, Molloy AR, Walker S, et al. The efficacy of intrathecal morphine and clonidine in the treatment of pain after spinal cord injury. Anesth Analg 2000;91(6):1493–8.
[68] Attal N, Gaude V, Brasseur L, et al. Intravenous lidocaine in central pain: a double-blind, placebo-controlled, psychophysical study. Neurology 2000;54(3):564–74.
[69] Chiou-Tan FY, Tuel SM, Johnson JC, et al. Effect of mexiletine on spinal cord injury dysesthetic pain. Am J Phys Med Rehabil 1996;75(2):84–7.
[70] Finnerup NB, Biering-Sorensen F, Johannesen IL, et al. Intravenous lidocaine relieves spinal cord injury pain: a randomized controlled trial. Anesthesiology 2005;102(5):1023–30.
[71] Loubser PG, Akman NM. Effects of intrathecal baclofen on chronic spinal cord injury pain. J Pain Symptom Manage 1996;12(4):241–7.
[72] Agency for Healthcare Research and Quality. Management of chronic central neuropathic pain following traumatic spinal cord injury. Summary, Evidence Report/Technology Assessment: Number 45. Rockville (MD): Agency for Healthcare Research and Quality; September 2001. AHRQ Publication Number 01–E062. Available at: http://www.ahrq.gov/clinic/epcsums/neurosum.htm. Accessed December 15, 2006.
[73] Putzke JD, Richards JS, Ness T, et al. Test-retest reliability of the Donovan spinal cord injury pain classification scheme. Spinal Cord 2003;41:239–41.
[74] Richards JS, Hicken BL, Putzke JD, et al. Reliability characteristics of the Donovan spinal cord injury pain classification system. Arch Phys Med Rehabil 2002;83:1290–4.
[75] Finnerup NB, Yezierski RP, Sang CN, et al. Treatment of spinal cord injury pain. Pain: Clinical Updates 2001;9(2):1–13.
[76] Siddall PJ, Middleton JW. A proposed algorithm for the management of pain following spinal cord injury. Spinal Cord 2005;44(2):67–77.
[77] Bryce TN, Ragnarsson KT. Pain after spinal cord injury. Phys Med Rehabil Clin N Am 2001;11(1):157–68.
[78] Finnerup NB, Johannesen IL, Sindrup SH, et al. Pharmacological treatment of spinal cord injury pain. In: Yezierski RP, Burchiel KJ, editors. Spinal cord injury pain: assessment, mechanisms, management. Seattle (WA): IASP Press; 2002. p. 341–51.
[79] Curtis KA, Tyner TM, Zachary L, et al. Effect of a standard exercise protocol on shoulder pain in long-term wheelchair users. Spinal Cord 1999;37:421–9.
[80] Cardenas DD, Warms CA, Turner JA, et al. Efficacy of amitriptyline for relief of pain in spinal cord injury: results of a randomized controlled trial. Pain 2002;96:365–73.
[81] Capel ID, Dorrell HM, Spencer EP, et al. The amelioration of the suffering associated with spinal cord injury with subperception transcranial electrical stimulation. Spinal Cord 2003; 41:109–17.
[82] Fregni F, Boggio PA, Lima MC, et al. A sham-controlled, phase II trial of transcranial direct current stimulation for the treatment of central pain in traumatic spinal cord injury. Pain 2006;122:197–209.
[83] Tan G, Rintala DH, Thornby JI, et al. Using cranial electrotherapy stimulation to treat pain associated with spinal cord injury. J Rehabil Res Dev 2006;43(4):461–74.
[84] Morley S, Eccleston C, Williams A. Systematic review and meta-analysis of randomized controlled trials of cognitive behaviour therapy and behaviour therapy for chronic pain in adults, excluding headache. Pain 1999;80(102):1–13.

[85] Ehde DM, Jensen MP. Feasibility of a cognitive restructuring intervention for treatment of chronic pain in persons with disabilities. Rehabil Psychol 2004;49(3):254–8.
[86] Gironda RJ. An interdisciplinary, cognitive-behavioral shoulder pain treatment program for individuals with paraplegia. SCI Psychosocial Process 2005;17(4):247–52.
[87] Norrbrink Budh C, Lund I, Ertzgaard P, et al. Pain in a Swedish spinal cord injury population. Clin Rehabil 2003;17:685–90.
[88] Jensen MP, Hanley MA, Engel JM, et al. Hypnotic analgesia for chronic pain in persons with disabilities: a case series. Int J Clin Exp Hypn 2005;53(2):198–228.
[89] Haythornthwaite JA, Wegener S, Benrud-Larson L, et al. Factors associated with willingness to try different pain treatments for pain after a spinal cord injury. Clin J Pain 2003; 19(1):31–8.
[90] Wegener ST, Shertzer E. Psychological Interventions in the management of SCI-related pain. Spinal Cord Inj Psych Proc 2005;17(4):238–46.
[91] ENRICHD. Enhancing recovery in coronary heart disease (ENRICHD) study intervention: rationale and design. Spinal Cord Injury Psychosocial Process 2001;63:747–55.
[92] Elliott TR, Shewchuck R. Using the nominal group technique to identify problems experienced by persons living with severe physical disabilities. J Clin Psychol Med Set 2002;9: 65–76.
[93] Elliott TR, Kennedy P. Treatment of depression following spinal cord injury: an evidence-based review. Rehabil Psychol 2004;49(2):134–9.
[94] Rehabilitation Accreditation Commission standards manual: medical rehabilitation, revised ed. Tucson (AZ): Rehabilitation Accreditation Commission; 2002.
[95] Flor H, Fydrich T, Turk DC. Efficacy of multidisciplinary pain treatment centers: a meta-analytic review. Pain 1992;49:221–30.

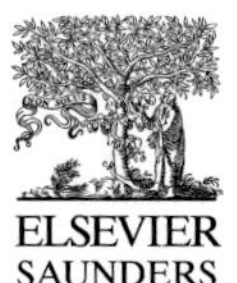

ELSEVIER
SAUNDERS

Phys Med Rehabil Clin N Am
18 (2007) 235–253

PHYSICAL MEDICINE AND REHABILITATION CLINICS OF NORTH AMERICA

The Prevention and Treatment of Pressure Ulcers

Chester H. Ho, MD[a,b,c,d,*], Kath Bogie, DPhil[c,d,e]

[a]*Spinal Cord Injury, Louis Stokes Cleveland Department of Veterans Affairs Medical Center, SCI 128W 10701 East Boulevard, Cleveland, OH 44106, USA*

[b]*Department of Physical Medicine & Rehabilitation, Case Western Reserve University, MetroHealth Medical Center, 2500 MetroHealth Drive, Cleveland, OH 44109, USA*

[c]*Cleveland Functional Electrical Stimulation Center, Louis Stokes Cleveland Department of Veterans Affairs Medical Center, SCI 128W 10701 East Boulevard, Cleveland, OH 44106, USA*

[d]*Advanced Platform Technology Center, Louis Stokes Cleveland Department of Veterans Affairs Medical Center, SCI 128W 10701 East Boulevard, Cleveland, OH 44106, USA*

[e]*Department of Orthopaedics, Case Western Reserve University, 10900 Euclid Ave., Cleveland, OH 44106, USA*

Pressure ulcers remain a significant secondary complication for many individuals with spinal cord injury (SCI). Technological advances in nonmedical fields, such as nanotechnology, are proceeding rapidly. Such hi-tech developments have the potential to affect both the prevention of future chronic wound development and the care of existing pressure ulcers. There is also a potential benefit in using developments that are initialized outside of the medical field, because high research and development costs are more readily absorbed by high-volume applications and may then be available at lower relative cost for comparatively low-volume medical care. For example, sensors developed for the automotive industry may have applications in the field of wound care.

The focus of this chapter is hi-tech devices and methodologies, which have the potential to have a significant impact on the field of pressure ulcer prevention and treatment. The current state-of-the-art methods are discussed with descriptions of currently available methods and research study findings. Conceptual approaches will also be presented, including

* Corresponding author. Spinal Cord Injury, Louis Stokes Cleveland Department of Veterans Affairs Medical Center, SCI 128W 10701 East Boulevard, Cleveland, OH 44106.

E-mail address: chester.ho@va.gov (C.H. Ho).

doi:10.1016/j.pmr.2007.02.004

therapeutic methods and devices that could become available in the next 5 to 10 years.

The options for pressure ulcer prevention are currently limited; however, as multidisciplinary approaches are integrated with improved clinical care, the potential impact of nontraditional approaches is great. There are many current options for treatment, and more continue to be developed that incorporate recent advances in fields such as biotechnology, imaging, and device design. In the current review, both the current state-of-the-art and conceptual approaches are discussed. Novel drug therapies are outside the scopes of this review and are not discussed.

Prevention of pressure ulcers

The assessment of techniques and devices to prevent pressure ulcer formation faces the challenges inherent in any attempt to determine the effectiveness of a prevention strategy. The initial basic research must develop efficacious techniques to reduce morbidity and improve quality of life. It is relatively straightforward to define the concept of pressure ulcer prevention as delaying or averting the development of a pressure ulcer. However, in practice, it is very difficult to objectively measure nonoccurrence of events without either controls or very large subject groups. Pressure ulcer development is known to be multifactorial, with applied pressure, duration of applied pressure, and blood flow (or tissue oxygenation) being among the primary factors. However, the relative weight of different factors has not been established fully. Surrogate indicators of changes in risk status may be used; however, care must be taken to ensure that outcomes measures are reliable, objective, and quantifiable.

Current state-of-the-art methods

Interface pressure mapping and monitoring of pressure ulcer risk status

Applied pressure has been used most frequently as a primary outcome measure in studies of devices, such as cushions, to prevent pressure ulcer development. The primary reason for this choice is pragmatic, namely that interface pressure mapping systems are widely available and established in both research and clinical settings.

The Skin Care Research Team (SCRT) at the Louis Stokes Cleveland DVA Medical Center has been investigating the use of a four-channel gluteal electrical stimulation system (GSTIM) to decrease risk factors associated with pressure ulcer development for individuals with SCI [1]. The semi-implanted system comprised implanted percutaneous electrodes together with an external stimulator. Assessment of seating posture was performed both during quiet sitting (static mode) and during use of the GSTIM system for weight shifting by alternate gluteal contractions (dynamic mode). To determine the sustained effects of long-term use of the

GSTIM system, repeated measures were made over a period of several months and years.

In this research study there was a requirement to monitor the effect of using the GSTIM system over time. Multiple outcomes measures were used, including interface pressure mapping. The research methodology has many similarities with the use of interface pressure mapping as an assessment tool in wheelchair and seating clinics [2,3]. In the clinic setting, patients often are evaluated several times, either on different cushions or over repeated visits to the clinic. There is a need to compare multiple assessments reliably using objective outcomes variables. To meet the research need in the GSTIM study, the Longitudinal Analysis with Self-Registration (LASR) statistical algorithm was developed to compare multiple pressure mapping datasets. This software tool also has the potential for widespread clinical implementation.

It is very challenging to ensure that the individual who is being assessed sits in exactly the same position at each assessment, particularly when assessments are at intervals of several weeks. In our research study, we were interested in both the short-term effects of GSTIM-induced weight shifting produced by alternating side-to-side gluteal contractions and the long-term effects of dynamic GSTIM use. It was therefore necessary to align pressure map images in both space (seated position) and time (phase of weight shifting).

The multistage LASR algorithm provides both spatial and temporal self-registration of pressure maps to allow comparison of repeated assessments over time for a single patient. The LASR output map shows the locations of statistically significant pressure changes across the entire mapped region without the requirement to predefine regions of interest. This allows clinicians and researchers to obtain more comprehensive, objective information including significantly different overall pressure distributions and the relative efficacy of pressure relief maneuvers. Output maps can be viewed as two-dimensional or three-dimensional "snapshots" of a single data frame or as movies (Fig. 1). Application of the LASR algorithm to paired pressure data sets requires a total processing time of 2 to 3 minutes after input of the raw data to production of the LASR output map, thus making it feasible for use in clinical settings.

LASR movies are particularly useful for determining the effectiveness of weight-shifting procedures; in our research study, weight-shifting was achieved using the GSTIM system. In the clinical setting, the efficacy of independent pressure relief procedures or dynamic cushions could be determined from LASR output movies. Examples can be found at http://stat.case.edu/lasr/. As seen in Fig. 1, the LASR algorithm showed that long-term use of the GSTIM system produced a significant decrease in ischial region seating interface pressures; these changes were sustained with routine daily GSTIM usage for more than 7 years in an individual with a C4 American Spinal Injury Association (ASIA) A tetraplegia [4].

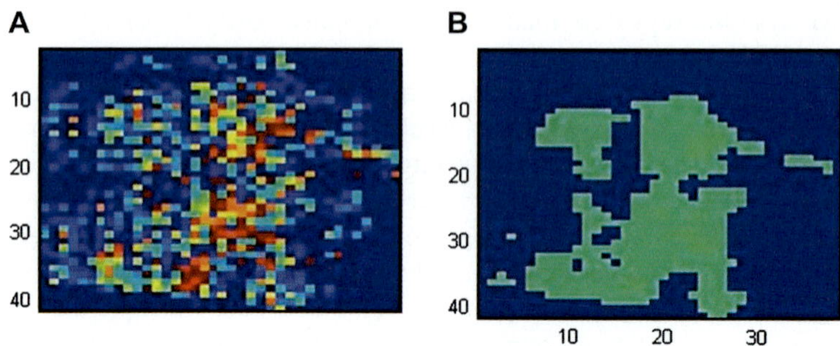

Fig. 1. LASR analysis maps for static mode seated pressure distributions showing areas of significant change over time for initial versus 40 months of daily GSTIM system use. The level of significance is adjusted for simultaneous testing at multiple locations. (*A*) Difference map. (*B*) LASR output (FDR P) map; significant differences are shown in green.

Dynamic pressure cushions and pressure alert systems

To minimize the risk of pressure ulcer development, a regime of regular pressure relief is essential. Adequate pressure relief can be achieved either by total removal of body weight from the loaded area or by weight-shifting to redistribute pressures. Individuals with spinal cord injury are recommended to change position every 2 hours when lying in bed and to perform pressure relief procedures every 15 to 20 minutes when seated in the wheelchair.

Individuals with impaired sensation and mobility often find it very hard to adhere to such a rigorous regime, because they do not feel pain or discomfort and also because they are unable to effectively weight-shift independently. For example, people with tetraplegia do not have sufficient upper body strength or trunk stability to perform independent pressure relief maneuvers. The current state-of-the-art method for independent pressure relief includes tilt-and-recline wheelchairs and dynamic pressure relief systems. There are a number of dynamic pressure-alternating support systems currently available commercially. The most options are available in alternating or low-air-loss mattresses. These devices are used routinely in many clinical settings and are considered both reliable and effective, although a recent Cochrane Report found that the relative merits of these hi-tech devices have not been clearly shown [5].

Dynamic wheelchair cushions may provide a means for reducing or varying interface pressures while seated. These devices work on the same principles as alternating pressure mattresses systems. In the past, alternating pressure cushions has not been as well embraced as a standard of care as mattresses. Early systems had many problems with reliability and were often too heavy for use in a manual wheelchair. Burns and Betz [6] reported that mean ischial region pressures were significantly lower with a dynamic wheelchair cushion during the low ischial pressure phase when compared with a gel cushion and tilted seating posture. However, there was little difference between the dynamic cushion and a dry flotation cushion with tilted posture.

Furthermore, the high ischial pressure phase produced higher mean regional pressures than either the gel or dry flotation cushion when seated upright in a tilt-in-space wheelchair.

Technological developments, including smaller, light-weight pumps and customization, have allowed some of these issues to be addressed. The USA Tech-Guide, produced by the United Spinal Association, currently lists more than 15 different powered alternating cushions from nine different manufacturers [7]. The majority of these cushions provide a regular pressure relief cycle of alternating rows or groups of cells inflating and deflating together. Pressure variation operates on a fixed cycle, typically of 4 to 5 minutes in duration. Some systems offer the capability to adjust "patient comfort level", ie, a subjective evaluation of acceptable inflation levels. Some cushions, such as the Ease Seating Systems (EASE Seating Systems, Paradise, California) can be tailored to individual requirements by adjusting cell layout. However, there is limited biofeedback or ability to vary factors such as cycle duration. Further research is needed to validate the efficacy and ease of use of dynamic wheelchair cushions before they can be universally accepted as a cost-effective approach to pressure ulcer prevention.

Individuals who are able to perform pressure relief maneuvers often find it difficult to adhere to a regular 20-minute regime, particularly when they have an active lifestyle and may have altered sensory function. For these individuals, a pressure relief reminder device may be highly beneficial and more economically viable than a dynamic wheelchair cushion. The design of such a device has been explored in preliminary feasibility studies in which the primary challenge was the design of an appropriate pressure sensor [8]. CleveMed (Cleveland, Ohio) has developed a patented biofeedback system, the Pressore Alert, which provides auditory or vibratory feedback to wheelchair users when pressure relief is necessary [9]. The device is programmable and can be set up to provide stimuli at appropriate time intervals, depending on the risk status and activity level of the individual.

Conceptual

Advances in early detection of pressure ulcers

Basic research studies are expanding knowledge of pressure ulcer etiology. For example, many clinicians have experienced the pressure ulcer that seems to "appear from nowhere"; one day the skin is mildly indurated but intact and the next there is a large open wound with extensive tissue breakdown and necrosis. There has been a growing clinical consensus that not all pressure ulcers are caused by high pressures at the skin interface and that deep tissue breakdown may be a significant factor in pressure ulcer development [10]. Several researchers have used finite element modeling and in vitro models to investigate the distribution of forces throughout the soft tissues. The research group at the Laboratory for Tissue Biomechanics and Engineering, Eindhoven University of Technology, The Netherlands has used a number of tissue muscle models to study the effects of applied strain and compressive forces on both the cellular level and on tissue constructs [11,12]. These studies found that the highest forces were experienced close to the bone interface. More recently, the group found the same force distributions in an animal model [13]. Furthermore, they found that short-term applied shear forces were much more causative of tissue damages than reversible ischemia. Animal model studies by Linder-Ganz and Geffen [14] also concluded that internal muscle stress is required to establish new criteria for pressure sore prevention.

These findings present a challenge to the clinician whose goal is the prevention of pressure ulcer development. At this time, there are limited techniques to monitor deep tissue viability. Any procedure to monitor tissue health to prevent pressure ulcer development would require regular assessment, ideally daily and at least weekly. Furthermore, at-risk individuals should be able to carry out the procedure with minimal disruption to their activities of daily living. Advanced imaging techniques, such as magnetic resonance imaging (MRI), have been used in research studies [15]. However, MRI evaluations clearly cannot meet the goals of a pressure ulcer prevention monitoring procedure. Daily, or even weekly, MRIs would be impractical and prohibitively expensive both for the health care system and the patient; indeed, in this scenario the cost of prevention may be greater than the cost of treatment.

The idea of nanotechnology was first introduced in the late 1950s by the renowned physicist, Richard Feynman [16]. Briefly, the concept is that of devices and materials being developed on the molecular scale, ie, of the order of 10^{-9} of a meter or 1 nanometer (nm). The associated field of microelectromechanical systems (MEMS) addresses the development of devices and materials with size from 10^{-6} of a meter (1 μm) to 10^{-3} of a meter (1 mm). Development in these fields has accelerated since the discovery of unique materials such as carbon nanotubes (buckytubes) and buckminsterfullerene (buckyballs). MEMS technology is moving out of the basic research laboratories and into mainstream application, such as automotive sensors and computer printers. In the medical field, BIOMEMS applications being developed include disposable blood pressure sensors and drug delivery systems.

Advances in the field of nanotechnology introduce the possibility of developing microscopically small devices. Nano devices, or nano-device arrays, could be implanted in the deep tissues of the high-risk individual with minimal disruption to the existing environment. These systems could provide real-time, in situ monitoring of biomechanical variables such as applied normal and shear forces, together with biochemical measures, such as temperature, pH, or lactate.

Other researchers have been investigating the role of biochemical indicators as precursors of pressure ulcer development. Bader and his group investigated early changes in the sweat metabolism of at-risk individuals during prolonged loading [17,18]. In their studies, a method for collection of sweat samples at discrete intervals was developed. Advances in the field of biosensors introduce the possibility of wearable devices for continuous monitoring. This approach is already being explored by the BIOTEX Project of the Sixth Framework Program of the European Commission [19]. The project goals include the development of a sensing patch on a textile substrate. The development of a smart textile for use in wheelchair or mattress covers would seem to be a highly attainable goal within the next 5 to 10 years.

Treatment of pressure ulcers

Current state-of-the-art methods

Novel treatment modalities: negative pressure wound therapy

Negative pressure wound therapy (NPWT) is based on the theory that the negative pressure generated drains wounds of exudates and enhances wound healing through a number of mechanisms [20]. More specifically, NPWT is proposed to decrease bacterial load and edema while concurrently promoting and improving local circulation and increasing granulation. The technique is also known as "subatmospheric pressure therapy," "vacuum sealing," "vacuum pack therapy," and "sealing aspirative therapy."

NWPT devices consist of a suction pump with foam and occlusive dressing to create negative pressure on the wounds that they are treating. The most common known NPWT device is probably "Vacuum Assisted Closure" (V.A.C.®), which was trademarked by Kinetics Concepts, Inc., San Antonio, TX (KCI) in 1997.

Although there are currently no official guidelines on the use of NPWT, the manufacturers have provided clinical guidelines for the use of the V.A.C.® device [21], and there have been recent consensus reports by Sibbald and colleagues [22] and Gupta [23]. The primary recommendations of these reports are that NPWT is indicated under the following clinical criteria:

- Anatomic surfaces that allow a tight seal.
- Adequately prepared wounds, eg, debrided, free of eschar and necrotic materials.
- Wound drainage.
- Patient compliance.

NPWT is contraindicated when wounds are dry, there is uncontrolled pain, there is untreated infection or malnutrition, or there is poor hemostasis.

Although there is no official guideline on NPWT device settings, the consensus reports recommended a negative pressure of 75 to 125 mm Hg. The precise pressure setting is dependent on the wound condition and the level of coexisting pain; it is recommended that a lower pressure be used if pain is an issue. Negative pressure should be applied continuously for the first 48 hours followed by intermittent negative pressure thereafter (5 minutes on, 2 minutes off). Effective NPWT will produce a response within 2 to 4 weeks.

Discontinuation is recommended if there is less than 30% wound size reduction after 4 weeks.

Despite its popularity, none of the major clinical reviews and guidelines has found sufficient scientific evidence to support the use of NPWT for wound healing. Over the period from 2000 to 2006, meta-analyses of clinical studies of NPWT have been performed by the Agency for Healthcare Research & Quality (AHRQ) [24], the Cochrane review [25], the Ministry of Health and Long-term Care of Ontario [26], the McGill University Health Center [27], and the PVA Consortium Clinical Practice Guideline panel [28]. There were several common reasons that these reports did not support the scientific basis of NPWT. It was universally found that there were too few randomized, controlled trials for NWPT. In addition, both small sample size and poor study design limited the validity of theses studies. Further research is needed to determine the utility of NPWT as a treatment modality for some nonhealing pressure ulcers. Currently, judicious use of NPWT should only be considered when performed under the auspices of the consensus reports discussed above.

Novel treatment modalities: pulsatile lavage therapy

Hydrotherapy is one of the two modalities recommended by the Agency for Health Care Policy and Research (AHCPR) for pressure ulcer management [29]. It is particularly helpful for cleansing and debridement of stage III and IV wounds. Conventionally, hydrotherapy for pressure ulcer management has been performed through the use of a whirlpool. However, the whirlpool has been found to have some clinical and practical limitations. Specifically;

- Cross-contamination between patients may occur, with multiple cases of pseudomonas infections being reported in the literature [30].
- The pressure jets may not be directed specifically at the pressure ulcers, thus the exact pressure applied to the wounds is not known.
- The cleansing and sterilization procedure may be rather cumbersome.
- Skin infections are potentially hazards for caregivers who are in contact with the contaminated water.

Other important issues are specific to individuals with spinal cord injury:

- It is very labor intensive to transfer the spinal cord–injured individuals with limited mobility into and out of the whirlpool.
- The sensory impairment in these individuals may result in burn injury if the water temperature is too high.
- Submersion into the whirlpool may affect body temperature control, especially for those with a higher level injury.

Therefore, despite the effectiveness of whirlpool therapy, it may not be ideal for use for individuals with spinal cord injury.

Pulsatile lavage therapy is a different form of hydrotherapy that encompasses all of the advantages of whirlpool therapy but without the potential adverse effects. A portable device is used that delivers pulsed jet streams of water at a known, preset pressure, which is compliant with the pressure range (4 to 15 psi) recommended for wound cleansing [31]. The device is for single-patient use only and is applied over the pressure ulcer, with the jet streams of water aiming directly into the wound bed through a soft, fan-spray tip. Some models also have concurrent suction that takes the soiled fluid back into a sealed collection canister, thus eliminating any significant spillage around the treatment area. The potential for cross-contamination between patients is eliminated because the device is for single-patient use and is used by a caregiver in the patient's room. In addition, there is no risk of any skin infection for the caregiver, provided that appropriate protective garments are being worn. However, the use of pulsatile lavage for multiple patients in the same location, without limiting the equipment for single-patient use, may lead to adverse outcomes with cross-contamination [32]. Because the treatment is localized to the wound area and uses a room temperature fluid, there is no risk for burn injury or any temperature dysregulation. Furthermore, pulsatile lavage therapy is less labor intensive than whirlpool hydrotherapy because it does not involve any transfer, and there is no cleansing of equipment afterward.

These factors also make pulsatile lavage appropriate for pressure ulcer debridement for home use [33]. Therefore, pulsatile lavage appears to be a preferred alternative to whirlpool therapy in the management of pressure ulcers. The clinical efficacy of pulsatile lavage in the treatment of pressure ulcers is currently under investigation.

Advances in pressure ulcer assessment: the use of telehealth for pressure ulcer management

The outpatient evaluation and monitoring of pressure ulcers in persons with spinal cord injury can be rather challenging at times because of the limited availability of appropriate transportation and poor pressure relief surface options while the individuals travel to see the evaluating clinician. The process of traveling to a clinical appointment could ironically pose more harm to the pressure ulcers to be evaluated. This process can present a dilemma to the clinician, who needs to balance the benefits of a pressure ulcer evaluation against the potential adverse effects of travel.

With the advances in technology, telehealth is becoming increasingly common and can provide us with the means to evaluate and monitor patients with pressure ulcers [34,35], while eliminating the need for long-distance travel. Telehealth is defined as long-distance communication between the patient and the health care provider via electronic means, such as video and audio. Studies have found that telehealth can provide accurate evaluation of wounds [36–38]. Telehealth can be used for pressure ulcer management and may be applied as home-based telehealth or clinic-to-clinic telehealth. In each case, the data delivery may be done immediately ("real-time") or be obtained and then delivered at a later time ("store-and-forward"). Both real-time and store-and-forward telehealth programs have been found to be accurate, although there is trade-off between cost and efficiency; the real-time system is more expensive to set up but clinically more efficient, whereas the store-and-forward system is less expensive to set up but less efficient [39].

Home-based telehealth can be used for the management of pressure ulcers by the transmission of digital images from the patient's home to the clinician's office, either through the use of a real-time video camera or through store-and-forward digital photography [40]. High-definition wound images can be sent over a regular telephone line, the internet [41], or even a wireless telephone [42,43]. For spinal cord–injured individuals, this may require the assistance of the caregivers to capture images and transmit them from home. In such cases, training of the caregiver will be necessary. Depending on the system and equipment used, there may or may not be direct interaction between the patients at home and the clinician in the clinic. The resolution of the images depends on the transmission speed of the equipment as well as the quality of the imaging device. There are currently no established standards for home-based devices and appropriate transmission speeds for the reliable evaluation of pressure ulcers using telehealth.

Clinic-to-clinic telehealth can provide subspecialty evaluation of pressure ulcers from one clinic to another [44]. The patients at the referral site are able to directly interact with the consultant through the real-time video. In addition to providing direct evaluation of pressure ulcers, clinic-to-clinic telehealth can also provide the means by which long-distance evaluation of other factors that affect pressure ulcer healing, including interface pressure measurement by pressure mapping, and seating or wheelchair evaluation. Our clinic at the Louis Stokes Cleveland DVA Medical Center has designed a dual screen system with one screen showing the posture of the patients at the referral site, while the other screen provides live data of pressure mapping from the referral site (Fig. 2). The clinic personnel at both the referral and consulting sites require training for the operation of the equipment, and a high-speed internet line is essential to provide high-resolution images and video. Using the clinic-to-clinic telehealth system, comprehensive pressure ulcer evaluations can now be done with the patients attending the local primary care clinic that would otherwise not have the special expertise for pressure ulcer management. Just as with home-based telehealth, there are currently no standards for devices and communication protocols to be used for clinic-to-clinic telehealth.

Using both home-based and clinic-to-clinic telehealth systems, pressure ulcers can be effectively and comprehensively managed over long distances. Participating patients no longer have to travel long distances for subspecialty care, thus improving the access to care for spinal cord–injured

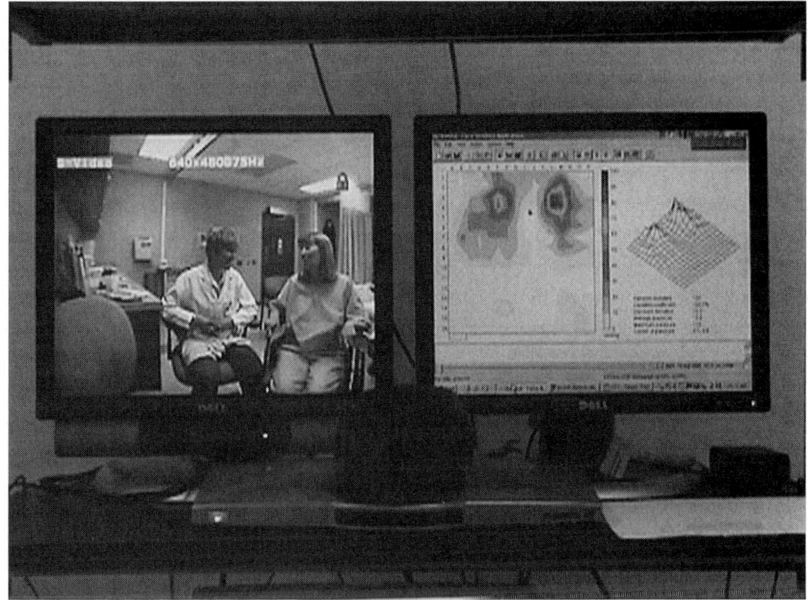

Fig. 2. Dual screen configuration for clinic-to-clinic real-time telehealth clinic.

individuals and avoiding any high costs associated with long distance travel. In addition, telehealth can provide educational training and help standardize care across a large geographical area united by a single telehealth network. It also enables the clinicians to provide teleconsultations to more patients than without the use of telehealth [45]. Currently, telehealth is not the standard of care in most geographical areas; however, it is expected to gain popularity as the technology becomes more affordable and available. The future growth of telehealth will be critically dependent on the resolution of important issues such as data security duration transmission and medicolegal concerns [46].

Advances in pressure ulcer assessment: the use of digital measurement techniques

Accurate wound measurement is of utmost importance in the monitoring and outcome evaluation of pressure ulcers in both clinical care and research. Over the last decade, wound evaluation tools have been developed that combine subjective assessment with wound size measurement [47,48]. A recent survey found that the majority of the surveyed clinicians felt that improvement is possible in the objective measurement of wound size [49]. Conventionally, linear measurements of length, width, and depth have been used widely in clinical care. However, this may not provide the most reliable evaluation, especially for pressure ulcers that are large, deep, and irregular in size and shape. Linear measures also tend to overestimate the surface area [50]. Furthermore, the linear measurements may have low interrater reliability. Assessment of wound healing over time incorporating repeated clinical evaluation together with reliable objective quantification of wound dimensions is essential to evaluate both current standards of care and new therapies. Therefore, alternative wound measurement methods that provide high accuracy and good interrater reliability would be very desirable. Digital wound measurement devices can potentially have these qualities that would be helpful in both the clinical and research settings.

Chronic wounds of varying etiologies can be highly variable in appearance and size. The ideal wound measurement technique would be able to accurately define the size of any wound, no matter what its depth, surface area, location, or the extent of undermining or tunneling. Critical geometric variables that could fully describe the wound "space" include maximum linear dimensions (length, width, and depth), aspect ratio, and circumference. In addition to providing an index of wound size, quantitative techniques must be reliable, repeatable, sensitive, and valid. The technology used must be robust and safe for both patients and clinical staff, cause no pain to the patient, and produce minimal additional disruption to ongoing care.

Two digital imaging techniques that have recently been introduced for clinical use may provide increased accuracy in determining linear wound dimensions and surface area. The Visitrak (Smith & Nephew, Largo, Florida) system represents a planimetry approach and requires wound contact for measurement. The VeV MD (Verge Videometer Measurement Documentation) system (Vistamedical, Manitoba, Canada) is a digital image analysis technique with photogrammetry that requires no contact for wound surface area measurement.

Visitrak is a tracing measurement technique that uses a transparent tracing film and a calculation tablet. The transparent, thin, flexible plastic sheet is placed over the wound area, and the outline is traced manually by the clinician using a permanent marker. The transparent film is then retraced on the Visitrak tablet. The Visitrak software then calculates the maximum length, width, and surface area of the traced wound automatically. Good inter- and intrarater reliability has been shown with this technique [51].

The VeV MD system is a noncontact technique based on the use of digital image analysis. It requires a digital photo of the wound with a standard target plate of known size to be placed next to the wound. After the images have been uploaded onto the computer, the outline of the wound's digitalized image is then traced manually by the clinician on the computer monitor. This area subsequently is compared with the adjacent standard target plate by the program's software, automatically calculating the surface area of the wound (Fig. 3). This measurement software has been used for the evaluation wound size in research studies [52].

In comparison with conventional linear measurements, these digital techniques have the advantage of measuring the actual surface area, rather than

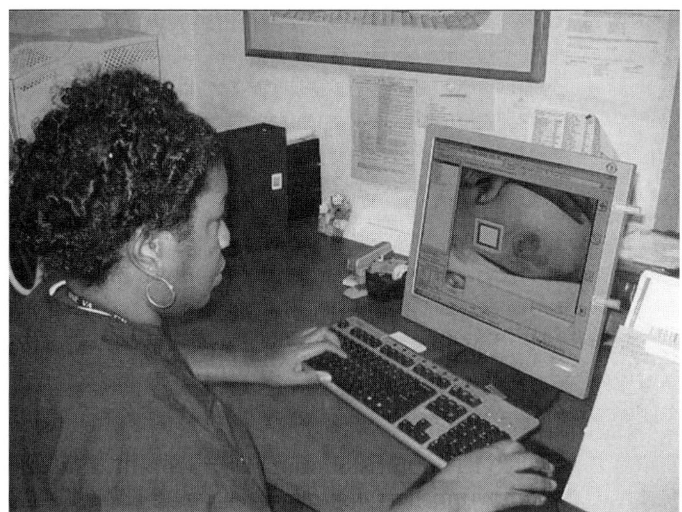

Fig. 3. VeV MD system in use.

surrogate measurements such as length and width. Both digital techniques were shown to have higher accuracy than linear measurement [53]. Furthermore, they may readily form part of an electronic record for the documentation of pressure ulcers. However, they do require an initial investment for the necessary equipment and software and training of the users. Furthermore, they may potentially consume more time than conventional measurements. None of these techniques measures the wound volume, which is the most accurate measurement for wound healing evaluation. All these factors need to be considered before deciding which measurement method would be the most appropriate for clinical or research purposes.

Conceptual

Advanced pressure ulcer imaging and measurement

The expansion of pressure ulcer measurement to fully visualize the three-dimensional (3-D) wound space will require the use of advanced imaging techniques and will incorporate technology from nonmedical fields. One example of this approach has been applied to development of a user-friendly device and software system to create quantified 3-D wound images.

Stereophotogrammetry is based on the ability to construct 3-D images from stereotactic 2-D images, ie, images of an object viewed from two slightly different angles can be combined to give a perception of depth. The application of this technique to wound measurement was first described by Bulstrode and colleagues [54] in 1986. The investigators evaluated both model wounds and clinical ulcers and found the technique to be highly accurate. Although the technique was quick and simple for the patient, subsequent image analysis required a high degree of observer training and was very slow and costly. This measurement technique used advanced optical principles to determine highly accurate measures of wound size; however, the technology to support optimal development of this approach was not available at that time, and it never became more than an interesting research tool.

Advances in digital technology and image analysis recently have led to the design of systems that may be applicable in both research and clinical applications. MAVIS-II (Measurement of Area and Volume Instrument System, University of Glamorgan, Wales) is a novel stereophotogrammetry system that combines standard off-the-shelf digital hardware with advanced image processing and measurement software to provide accurate multidimensional wound measurement [55]. MAVIS-II hardware comprises a standard digital camera (4 megapixels or greater) together with a stereophotogrammetric adapter. The MAVIS-II system can measure wound dimensions rapidly and without physical contact. The system incorporates a simple light-calibration mechanism for ensuring the camera is a standard distance from the wound at each assessment. The system is portable ands easy to use with a reported precision of about 5% in all linear dimensions (length, width, and depth). MAVIS-II wound images are produced in 3-D (Fig. 4) and can be rotated on the screen to give a fuller view of varying wound depth (for an example, see: http://www.medimaging.org/mavis).

Pressure ulcer treatment without bed rest

For many individuals in whom pressure ulcers develop, the requirement for continuous bed rest is onerous and highly detrimental to their quality of life. Moreover, it can negatively affect other aspects of their clinical condition, such as respiratory function and functional abilities. In addition, financial limitations on rehabilitation coverage often dictate that patients with pressure ulcers be mobilized early.

Options to treat or manage pressure ulcers without bed rest are thus of interest to the patient, clinical team, and insurance companies. One traditional approach has been to use prone trolleys, with which patients can gain some mobility, but the prone position is limited in function.

Over the last decade, standing wheelchairs have become an increasingly popular option for independent mobility. These systems can be used to provide a full, extended pressure relief over pelvic region wounds, thus allowing remobilization of individuals with existing pressure ulcers. Standing wheelchairs also have benefits in addition to pressure ulcer treatment. Dunn and colleagues [56] in a 1998 survey of 99 standing wheelchair users found that the patients reported improvements in lower extremity range of motion, upper extremity strength, and bladder and other systemic functions together with decreased spasm and pain.

The USA Tech-Guide lists over 15 power standing wheelchairs and 11 manual standing wheelchairs [57,58]. The Independence® iBOT® 4000

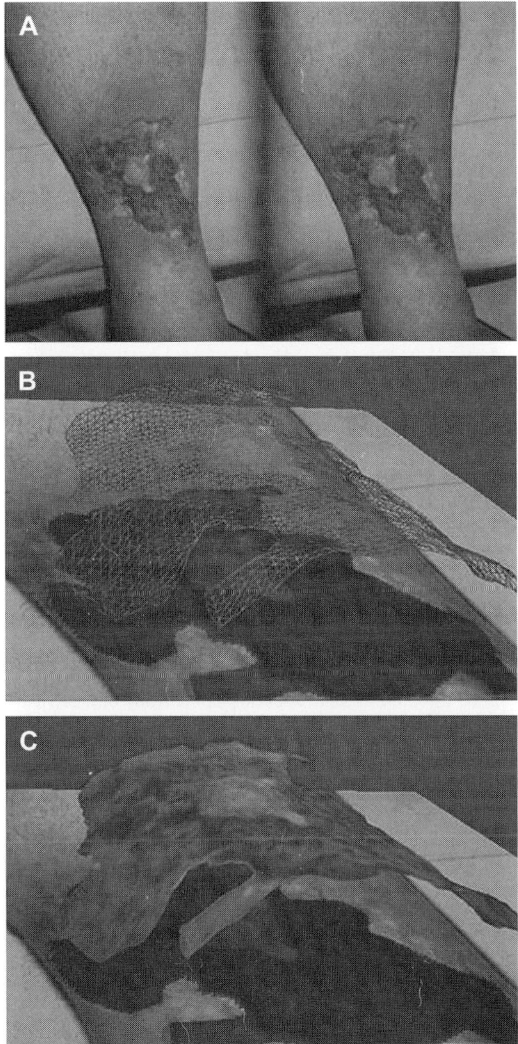

Fig. 4. MAVIS wound analysis output. Courtesy of P. Plassmann, PhD, University of Glamorgan, Wales. (*A*) Source stereo images of wound. (*B*) 3-D mesh of wound. (*C*) 3-D model of wound.

Mobility System (Endicott, NY) currently is the most advanced power standing wheelchair available. It allows users to mobilize while standing and to climb curbs and steps without assistance. However, this broad-ranging functionality is costly and thus currently inaccessible for most people with SCI. The Veterans Administration has instigated a program whereby veterans with SCI may be eligible for receive an iBOT® system dependent on rigorous guidelines that include an extensive clinical evaluation.

An alternative approach to a full standing wheelchair is to vary individual system components to relieve pressure over areas of tissue breakdown. Mahkous's group at the Rehabilitation Institute of Chicago are investigating the use of wheelchair in which ischial region pressures are varied by movement of the rear portion of the seat base [59]. The group found that sitting with decreased ischial support and a fitted lumbar backrest minimized posterior sacral rotation and transferred seating pressures from the ischial region forward to the thigh region.

Little research exists to validate the use of dynamic wheelchair cushions for the treatment of pressure ulcers. However, the benefits would be similar to those achieved using a standing or dynamically variable wheelchair system. Technologically advanced devices, such as the Airpulse PK (Aquila Corporation, La Crosse, Wisconsin), can be tailored to the individual requirements by adjusting inflation levels, cycle time, cycling action, and customizing cell layout.

Further research is needed to determine the relative merits of dynamic wheelchairs, standing wheelchairs, and dynamic wheelchair cushions for pressure ulcer treatment based on multidisciplinary clinical and health services outcomes measures.

References

[1] Bogie KM, Reger SI, Levine SP. Therapeutic applications of electrical stimulation; wound healing and pressure sore prevention. Assist Technol 2000;12:50–66.

[2] Sprigle S. Interface pressure measurement: applying research findings to clinical use. Proceedings of the RESNA 26th International Conference on Technology and Diversity, Atlanta (GA); 2003.

[3] Crawford SA, Strain B, Gregg B, et al. An investigation of the impact of the Force Sensing Array pressure mapping system on the clinical judgement of occupational therapists. Clin Rehabil 2005;19:224–31.

[4] Bogie KM, Wang X, Triolo RJ. Long-term prevention of pressure ulcers in high-risk patients: a single case study of the use of gluteal neuromuscular electric stimulation. Arch Phys Med Rehabil 2006;87:585–91.

[5] Cullum N, McInnes E, Bell-Syer SE, et al. Support surfaces for pressure ulcer prevention. Cochrane Database Syst Rev 2004;3:CD001735.

[6] Burns SP, Betz KL. Seating pressures with conventional and dynamic wheelchair cushions in tetraplegia. Arch Phys Med Rehabil 1999;80(5):566–71.

[7] United Spinal Association, 2007. USA-TechGuide, A web guide to wheelchairs and assistive technology. Available at: http://www.usatechguide.org/reviews.php?vmode=1&catid=66. Accessed February 9, 2007.

[8] Cremar A, Reed G, Wang L. Design of a wheelchair pressure relief timer. Senior design project. Department of Bioengineering. University Park, PA: Pennsylvania State University, 2006.

[9] Cleveland Medical Devices Inc., 2004. Pressore Alert™. Available at: http://www.clevemed.com/prod_descriptions/pressorealert.htm. Accessed February 9, 2007.

[10] Black JM. National Pressure Ulcer Advisory Panel. Moving toward consensus on deep tissue injury and pressure ulcer staging. Adv Skin Wound Care 2005;18(8):415–6, 418, 420–1.

[11] Bouten CV, Breuls RG, Peeters EA, et al. In vitro models to study compressive strain-induced muscle cell damage. Biorheology 2003;40(1–3):383–8.

[12] Breuls RG, Bouten CV, Oomens CW, et al. A theoretical analysis of damage evolution in skeletal muscle tissue with reference to pressure ulcer development. J Biomech Eng 2003; 125(6):902–9.
[13] Stekelenburg A, Strijkers GJ, Parusel H, et al. The role of ischemia and deformation in the onset of compression-induced deep tissue injury: MRI-based studies in a rat model. J Appl Physiol 2007; [Epub ahead of print].
[14] Linder-Ganz E, Gefen A. Mechanical compression-induced pressure sores in rat hindlimb: muscle stiffness, histology, and computational models. J Appl Physiol 2004;96(6):2034–49 [Epub 2004 Feb 6].
[15] Linder-Ganz E, Shabshin N, Itzchak Y, et al. Assessment of mechanical conditions in sub-dermal tissues during sitting: A combined experimental-MRI and finite element approach. J Biomech 2006; [Epub ahead of print].
[16] Feynman RP. There's Plenty of Room at the Bottom. Available at: http://www.zyvex.com/nanotech/feynman.html. Accessed February 9, 2007.
[17] Polliack A, Taylor R, Bader D. Sweat analysis following pressure ischaemia in a group of debilitated subjects. J Rehabil Res Dev 1997;34(3):303–8.
[18] Knight SL, Taylor RP, Polliack AA, et al. Establishing predictive indicators for the status of loaded soft tissues. J Appl Physiol 2001;90(6):2231–7.
[19] Biotex Consortium, 2005. Bio-sensing textile for health management. Available at: http://www.biotex-eu.com. Accessed February 9, 2007.
[20] Morris GS, Brueilly KE, Hanzelka H. Negative pressure wound therapy achieved by vacuum-assisted closure: evaluating the assumptions. Ostomy Wound Manage 2007;53(1): 52–7.
[21] The Vacuum assisted closure (V.A.C.) therapy clinical guidelines. A reference source for clinicians; 2005. Available at: http://www.kci1.com/2-B-128_Clin_Guidelines_Blue_Book_1-05.pdf
[22] Sibbald RG, Mahoney J, V.A.C. Therapy Canadian Consensus Group. A consensus report on the use of vacuum-assisted closure in chronic, difficult-to-heal wounds. Ostomy Wound Manage 2003;49(11):52–66.
[23] Gupta S. Guidelines for managing pressure ulcers with negative pressure wound therapy. Adv Skin Wound Care 2004;17(Suppl 2):1–16.
[24] Samson D, Lefevre F, Aronson N. Wound healing technologies: low-level laser and vacuum-assisted closure. Evid Rep Technol Assess (Summ) 2004 Dec;111:1–6.
[25] Evans D, Land L. Topical negative pressure for treating chronic wounds. The Cochrane Institute of Systematic Reviews 2006;3.
[26] Vacuum assisted closure therapy for wound care. Health technology literature review. Toronto; December 2004. The Medical Advisory Secretariat, Ministry of Health and Long-Term Care.
[27] Costa V, Brophy J, McGregor M. Vacuum-assisted wound closure therapy (V.A.C.®). McGill University Health Centre; 2005. Report Number 19.
[28] Consortium for Spinal Cord Medicine Clinical Practice Guidelines. Pressure ulcer prevention and treatment following spinal cord injury: a clinical practice guideline for health-care professionals. Paralyzed Veterans of America 2000.
[29] Bergstrom N, Allman RM, Alvarez OM, et al. Treatment of pressure ulcers. Clinical practice guideline, Number 15. Rockville (MD): Agency for Health Care Policy and Research, Public Health Service, U.S. Department of Health and Human Services; 1994. AHCPR Publication No. 95–0652.
[30] Hollyoak V, Allison D, Summers J. Pseudomonas aeruginosa wound infection associated with a nursing home's whirlpool bath. Commun Dis Rep CDR Rev 1995;5(7):R100–2.
[31] Folkedahl BA, Frantz R. Treatment of pressure ulcers. Iowa City (IA): University of Iowa Gerontological Nursing Interventions Research Center, Research Dissemination Core; 2002. p. 30.

[32] Maragakis LL, Cosgrove SE, Song X, et al. An outbreak of multidrug-resistant Acinetobacter baumannii associated with pulsatile lavage wound treatment. JAMA 2004;292(24): 3006–11.
[33] Morgan D, Hoelscher J. Pulsed lavage: promoting comfort and healing in home care. Ostomy Wound Manage 2000;46(4):44–9.
[34] Mathewson C, Adkins VK, Jones ML. Initial experiences with telerehabilitation and contingency management programs for the prevention and management of pressure ulceration in patients with spinal cord injuries. J Wound Ostomy Continence Nurs 2000;27(5):269–71.
[35] Vesmarovich S, Walker T, Hauber R, et al. Use of telerehabilitation to manage pressure ulcers in persons with spinal cord injuries. Adv Wound Care 1999;12:264–9.
[36] Gardner SE, Frantz RA, Specht JK, et al. How accurate are chronic wound assessments using interactive video technology? J Gerontol Nurs 2001;27(1):52–3 [quiz: 15–20].
[37] Salmhofer W, Hofmann-Wellenhof R, Gabler G, et al. Wound teleconsultation in patients with chronic leg ulcers. Dermatology 2005;210:211–7.
[38] Halstead L, Dang T, Elrod M, et al. Teleassessment compared with live assessment of pressure ulcers in a wound clinic: a pilot study. Adv Skin Wound Care 2003;16:91–6.
[39] Loane MA, Bloomer SE, Corbett R, et al. A comparison of real-time and store-and-forward teledermatology: a cost-benefit study. Br J Dermatol 2000;143(6):1241–7.
[40] Lowery JC, Hamill JB, Wilkins EG, et al. Technical overview of a web-based telemedicine system for wound assessment. Adv Skin Wound Care 2002;15(4):165–6, 168–9.
[41] Kinsella A. Advanced telecare for wound care delivery. Home Healthc Nurse 2002;20(7): 457–61. Erratum in: Home Healthc Nurse 2002;20(8):537.
[42] Braun R, Vecchietti J, Thomas L, et al. Telemedicine wound care using a new generation of mobile telephones: a feasibility study. Arch Dermatol 2005;141(2):254–8.
[43] Hsieh CH, Tsai HH, Yin JW, et al. Teleconsultation with the mobile camera-phone in digital soft-tissue injury: a feasibility study. Plast Reconstr Surg 2004;114(7):1776–82.
[44] Ratliff C, Forch W. Telehealth for wound management in long-term care. Ostomy Wound Manage 2005;51(9):40–5.
[45] Kobza L, Scheurich A. The impact of telemedicine on outcomes of chronic wounds in the home care setting. Ostomy Wound Manage 2000;46(10):48–53.
[46] Jones S, Banwell P, Shakespeare P. Telemedicine in wound healing. Int Wound J 2004;1(4): 225–30.
[47] Stotts NA, Rodeheaver GT, Thomas DR, et al. An instrument to measure healing in pressure ulcers: development and validation of the pressure ulcer scale for healing (PUSH). J Gerontol A Biol Sci Med Sci 2001;56(12):M795–9.
[48] Woodbury MG, Houghton PE, Campbell KE, et al. Development, validity, reliability, and responsiveness of a new leg ulcer measurement tool. Adv Skin Wound Care 2004;17(4 Pt 1): 187–96.
[49] Berlowitz DR, Ratliff C, Cuddigan J, et al. The PUSH tool: a survey to determine its perceived usefulness. Adv Skin Wound Care 2005;18(9):480–3.
[50] Flanagan M. Improving accuracy of wound measurement in clinical practice. Ostomy Wound Manage 2003;49(10):28–40.
[51] Gethin G, Cowman S. Wound measurement comparing the use of acetate tracings and Visitrak digital planimetry. J Clin Nurs 2006;15(4):422–7.
[52] Thawer HA, Houghton PE, Woodbury MG, et al. A comparison of computer-assisted and manual wound size measurement. Ostomy Wound Manage 2002;48(10):46–53.
[53] Haghpanah S, Bogie K, Wang X, et al. Reliability of electronic versus manual wound measurement techniques. Arch Phys Med Rehabil 2006;87(10):1396–402.
[54] Bulstrode CJ, Goode AW, Scott PJ. Stereophotogrammetry for measuring rates of cutaneous healing: a comparison with conventional techniques. Clin Sci (Lond) 1986;71(4):437–43.
[55] Plassmann P, Jones TD. MAVIS: a non-invasive instrument to measure area and volume of wounds. Measurement of Area and Volume Instrument System. Med Eng Phys 1998;20(5): 332–8.

[56] Dunn RB, Walter JS, Lucero Y, et al. Follow-up assessment of standing mobility device users. Assist Technol 1998;10(2):84–93.
[57] United Spinal Association, 2007. Standing Wheelchairs → Manual Standing Wheelchairs. Available at: http://www.usatechguide.org/reviews.php?vmode=1&catid=98. Accessed February 9, 2007.
[58] United Spinal Association, 2007. Standing Wheelchairs → Power Standing Wheelchairs. Available at: http://www.usatechguide.org/reviews.php?vmode=1&catid=296. Accessed February 9, 2007.
[59] Makhsous M, Lin F, Hendrix RW, et al. Sitting with adjustable ischial and back supports: biomechanical changes. Spine 2003;28(11):1113–21 [discussion: 1121–2].

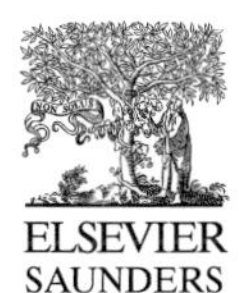

ELSEVIER
SAUNDERS

Phys Med Rehabil Clin N Am
18 (2007) 255–274

PHYSICAL MEDICINE
AND REHABILITATION
CLINICS OF
NORTH AMERICA

Neurogenic Bladder in Spinal Cord Injury

Gregory Samson, MD[a,b],
Diana D. Cardenas, MD, MHA[a,c,*]

[a]*Department of Rehabilitation Medicine, Leonard M. Miller School of Medicine, P.O. Box 016960 (D-461), Miami, FL 33101, USA*
[b]*Department of Veterans Affairs, Miami VA Healthcare System, Spinal Cord Injury Service (128), 1201 NW 16th Street, Miami, FL 33125, USA*
[c]*Miami Project to Cure Paralysis, Lois Pope LIFE Center, 1095 NW 14th Terrace, Miami, FL 33136, USA*

The bladder has two main functions: the storage of urine under low intravesical pressure and periodic release of urine in a controlled coordinated manner during an acceptable time to void. The ability to maintain continence and release urine is under voluntary control mediated by neural input to the lower urinary tract (LUT) from centers located in the brain and spinal cord. A neurogenic bladder dysfunction is the result of disease or injury to the neural pathways or neuromuscular junctions controlling LUT functions, and commonly occurs after spinal cord injury (SCI).

In the past, renal failure was the leading cause of death after SCI [1,2]. Today mortality from SCI has declined dramatically partly owing to the improved management of urologic dysfunction associated with SCI [3]. The goals of bladder management in SCI patients are intended to (1) ensure social continence for reintegration into community, (2) allow low-pressure storage and efficient bladder emptying at low detrusor pressures, (3) avoid stretch injury from repeated overdistension, (4) prevent upper and lower urinary tracts complications from high intravesical pressures, and (5) prevent recurrent urinary tract infections. This article provides an overview of neurogenic bladder dysfunction associated with SCI and current management options.

* Corresponding author. Department of Rehabilitation Medicine, University of Miami, Leonard M. Miller School of Medicine, P.O. Box 016960 (D-461), Miami, FL 33101.

E-mail address: dcardenas@med.miami.edu (D.D. Cardenas).

1047-9651/07/$ - see front matter
doi:10.1016/j.pmr.2007.03.005

Lower urinary tract anatomy and physiology

The LUT comprises the fundus, trigone, and neck of the bladder, the pelvic diaphragm, and the urethra. The bladder outlet consists of the bladder neck and urethral smooth and striated muscles. The urinary bladder is a four-layered musculomembranous structure composed primarily of smooth muscle cells that can contract when stretched. The four layers consist of (1) a three-layered detrusor muscle; (2) a serous layer; (3) a submucous, areolar layer; and (4) a thin mucous layer continuous with the ureteral and urethral linings. The structures primarily involved in the performance of bladder functions include the muscle of the fundus, bladder neck muscles, urethral smooth muscles, periurethral striated sphincter muscles, and striated pelvic muscles. The LUT urothelium acts as an active barrier, performing specialized sensory and signaling functions to regulate the chemical and physical environment.

Lower urinary tract innervation

Activity of the LUT must be coordinated during its storage and voiding phases. In the normally functioning LUT, the bladder outlet relaxes and bladder smooth muscle contracts during voiding while during the storage phase the detrusor relaxes and bladder neck contracts. Normal regulation of LUT functions is under voluntary control and involves a complex interplay between central and peripheral nervous system inputs (Fig. 1).

Peripheral innervation

Peripheral nervous system innervations include autonomic (sympathetic and parasympathetic) and somatic pathways (Fig. 1). Parasympathetic innervation provides excitation to the smooth muscle of the bladder and inhibitory input to the urethral sphincter smooth muscle. Fibers originate from preganglionic cholinergic neurons in the intermediolateral region at the sacral levels, S2 through S4 of the spinal cord. Axons then travel by way of the pelvic nerves to ganglionic cells within the pelvic plexus and bladder wall. Excitatory transmission to the bladder wall is mediated mostly through the action of acetylcholine on the M3 muscarinic receptor subtype [4]. The parasympathetic inhibitory input to the urethral sphincter, however, is mediated by the release of nitric oxide [5].

Sympathetic innervation provides inhibitory input to the bladder smooth muscle, excitation to the bladder neck, and modulation of parasympathetic ganglionic activity to the bladder. Thoracolumbar sympathetic pathways and prevertebral inferior mesenteric ganglia (T10–L2) travel primarily by way of the hypogastric nerves and also through the pelvic nerves. Noradrenaline release mediates inhibitory activity through β-adrenergic receptors on the bladder wall, whereas excitatory input to the bladder neck and urethra is through α1- and α2-adrenergic receptors [5].

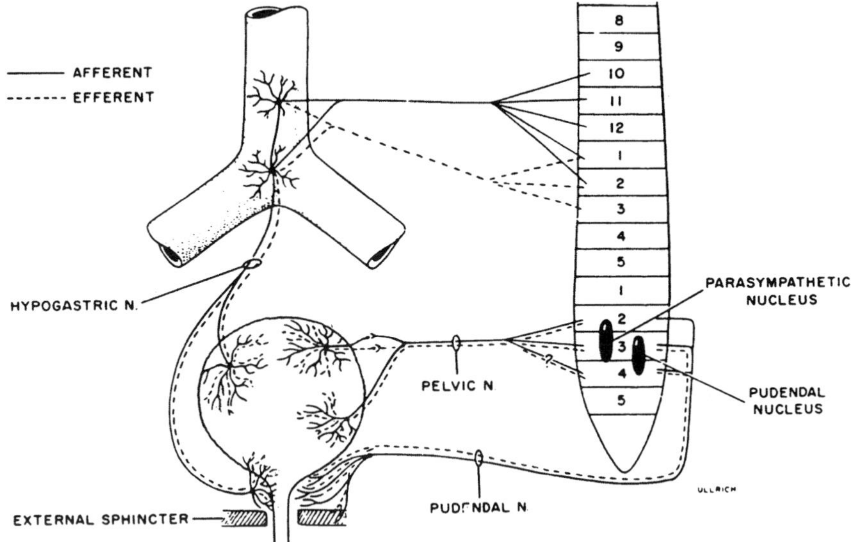

Fig. 1. The parasympathetic, sympathetic, and somatic nerve supply to the bladder, urethra, and pelvic floor. (*From* Cardenas DD, Mayo ME, King JC. Urinary tract and bowel management in the rehabilitation setting. In: Braddom RL, Buschbacher RM, Dumitru D, et al, editors. Physical medicine and rehabilitation. Philadelphia: W.B. Saunders; 1996. p. 555–79; with permission.)

Somatic efferent (motor) innervation from the Onuf's nucleus in the anterolateral horn of the sacral spinal cord, S2 through S3, provides excitatory input to the striated muscles of the urethral sphincter. The efferent fibers travel by way of the pudendal nerves to reach the urethral sphincter, and excitatory activity is mediated by acetylcholine action on nicotinic receptors. LUT sensory (afferent) impulses that are conveyed to the central nervous system arise from receptors in the bladder and urethra. Impulses travel along the pelvic nerves and sacral spinal cord mainly by way of small myelinated (A-δ) and unmyelinated (C) fibers. The A-δ fibers have mostly mechanoreceptor functions responding to tension, whereas C-fibers have mostly chemoreceptor functions, responding to inflammatory or noxious stimuli within the LUT [6]. Micturition is generally initiated through gradual bladder distension and contraction triggering the sensation of bladder filling and leading to A-δ afferent activation and subsequent active bladder contraction.

Central nervous system innervation

Voluntary control of voiding arises from the central nervous system, with centers located in both the brain and the spinal cord (Fig. 2). Spinal cord pathways include efferent neurons, interneurons, and afferent neurons. Afferent fibers from the urinary bladder and urethra project to interneurons

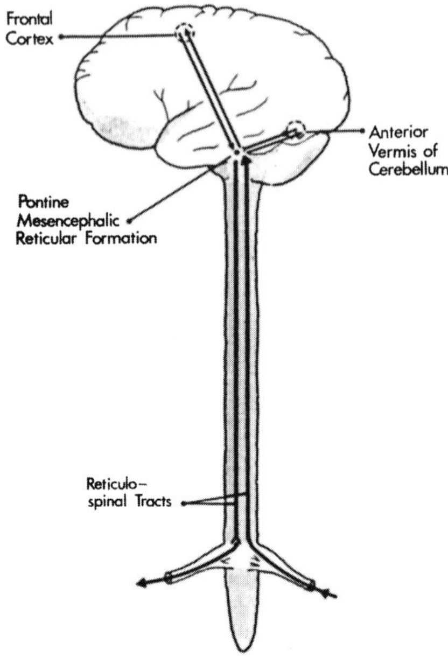

Fig. 2. The central connections of the bladder reflex are shown with the afferents ascending possibly in the reticulospinal tracts or the posterior columns to the pontine mesencephalic reticular formation, and the efferents running down to the sacral outflow in the reticulospinal tracts. The pontine center is largely influenced by the cortex but also by other areas of the brain, particularly the cerebellum and basal ganglia. (*From* Cardenas DD, Mayo ME, King JC. Urinary tract and bowel management in the rehabilitation setting. In: Braddom RL, Buschbacher RM, Dumitru D, et al, editors. Physical medicine and rehabilitation. Philadelphia: W.B. Saunders; 1996. p. 555–79; with permission.)

at the dorsal horn in the sacral spinal cord. Local connections involved in segmental spinal reflexes occur at that level. Other projections ascend through different pathways in the spinal cord to the pontine micturition center (PMC), periaqueductal gray matter, or ventral posterior nucleus of the thalamus and ultimately extend to the cerebral cortex.

Numerous other regions in the brain are believed to be involved in LUT control, including the medullary raphe nuclei, the locus coeruleus, the paraventricular nucleus of the hypothalamus, and neurons in the anterior hypothalamus [7]. Efferent information from these suprapontine regions, including the frontal cortex and periaqueductal gray matter, then project to the PMC which functions as the site of integration of supraspinal input to regulate reflex micturition at the spinal level. Efferent pathways originating from the PMC then project to (1) motor neurons innervating the external urethral sphincter that originate from Onuf's nucleus, (2) sacral parasympathetic preganglionic fibers, and (3) rostral lumbar sympathetic preganglionic fibers.

Normal micturition reflex

Normal bladder functions of storage and voiding are controlled by voluntary and reflex mechanisms. During the storage phase, the bladder must be able to expand slowly at low pressure until an appropriate bladder volume is reached, Sphincter activity must also be coordinated with bladder filling to allow adequate storage. Once threshold bladder volume is reached, the sacral reflex centers at S2 through S4 are stimulated with subsequent impulses sent from sacral spinal cord up to the PMC and frontal cortex. Efferent impulses sent from the brain stem stimulate bladder contraction, coordinated bladder neck relaxation, and closure of the ureteral valves, resulting in a sensation to void. If deemed socially appropriate, a conscious decision to void is initiated under the voluntary control of the frontal cortex which sends regulatory impulses to the external sphincter, by way of the corticospinal tract to the pudendal nerves. Voiding involves bladder wall contraction and relaxation of the internal and external sphincters. Conversely, if voiding is to be delayed, voluntary tightening of the external sphincter leads to associated bladder wall relaxation, internal sphincter contraction, and additional urine storage.

During the storage phase of bladder function, a sympathetic reflex activity through a local sacrolumbar spinal reflex pathway is triggered by afferent impulses in the pelvic nerves [8]. This negative feedback mechanism contributes to the storage function of the bladder by increasing urethral outflow resistance, increasing bladder capacity, and decreasing the frequency and amplitude of bladder contractions. Once a threshold for bladder pressure is reached, a supraspinal inhibitory response, likely originating from the PMC, suppresses the vesicosympathetic reflex pathway and allows micturition to occur. As the bladder fills, afferent input from the bladder along with bulbospinal pathways from the pons maintain the normal, coordinated relationship between bladder and sphincter [9]. This process further mediates activities of the striated muscles of the urethral sphincter and facilitates further bladder storage.

With voiding, afferent activity arising from tension receptors in the bladder activates neurons in the brainstem, the PMC, which functions as an "on/off" switch [10]. Neuronal pathways between the rostral brain and pons then provide regulatory input through the brainstem, which then provides parasympathetic control of micturition through activation of sacral parasympathetic efferent pathways to the bladder and urethra.

Classification of neurogenic bladder in spinal cord injury

Many classification systems pertaining to neurogenic bladder have been devised. It has generally been classified based on neurologic, neurourologic, and functional classifications. The neurologic classification devised by Bors and Comarr [11] can be applied to traumatic SCI. In this classification system, lesions are classified as either upper or lower motor neuron with respect to the anatomic location of the lesion relative to the sacral cord reflex centers.

Lower motor neuron

A lower motor neuron lesion is one that occurs at or below the conus medullaris (Fig. 3). These lesions can affect efferent (motor), afferent (sensory), or both portions of the sacral arc pathway. Classic findings include an areflexic or hyporeflexic detrusor with a normal or underactive external sphincter. With a denervated or underactive external sphincter, coordination between detrusor contraction and sphincter relaxation occurs during bladder emptying (no detrusor–external sphincter dyssynergia [DESD]). If all the peripheral fibers below the level of injury are affected, loss of sacral reflexes occurs along with an areflexic bladder (a so-called "complete injury"). If, however, only some of the peripheral fibers are intact, a sacral reflex may be present with an areflexic bladder, suggesting an incomplete injury lower motor neuron lesion involving the conus, cauda equina, or peripheral nerve.

In a motor (efferent) neurogenic bladder, supraspinal regulatory transmission to afferent sacral nerves is spared, leading to preserved sensation of fullness, although normal sensation may be gradually lost because of recurrent overdistension injury. With strictly sensory (afferent) lesions, patients are able to void but have decreased sensation, which can lead to chronic overdistension and impaired emptying. Lesions involving motor and sensory pathways (the most typical) are associated with a mixture of symptoms. In a complete lesion at or below the conus medullaris, urodynamic studies will show an areflexic, low-pressure detrusor, absent EMG activity, elevated postvoid residual; and a competent bladder outlet.

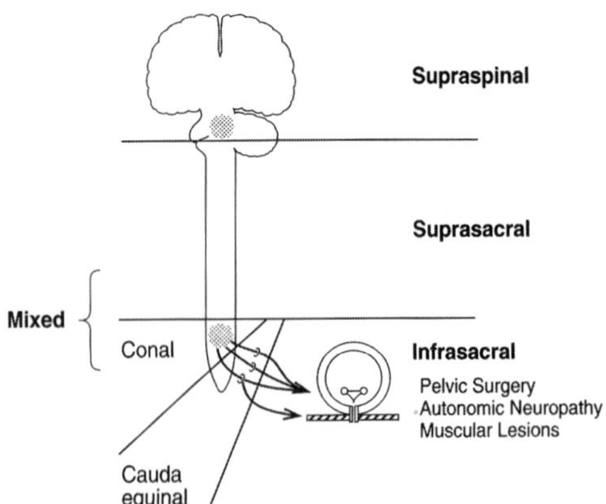

Fig. 3. Anatomic classification of the neurogenic bladder. (*From* Cardenas DD, Mayo ME, King JC. Urinary tract and bowel management in the rehabilitation setting. In: Braddom RL, Buschbacher RM, Dumitru D, et al, editors. Physical medicine and rehabilitation. Philadelphia: W.B. Saunders; 1996. p. 555–79; with permission.)

Upper motor neuron

Upper motor neuron lesions can be of two types: (1) intracranial (supra-pontine) lesions in which cortical input that inhibits detrusor contractility is interrupted while the PMC is intact, and (2) spinal (suprasacral or infrapontine) lesions pertaining to spinal cord injuries (Fig. 3). Spinal lesions occur above the conus medullaris and spare the sacral reflex arc. The descending pontine (central) modulation of detrusor and sphincter activity is therefore disrupted, leading to DESD; detrusor–internal sphincter dyssynergia may also occur in lesions above T6.

Because sacral reflexes are present, independent sacral reflex activity leads to uninhibited bladder contraction during filling at a given volume threshold, and urinary incontinence with no sensation of bladder filling or urge to void. Additional findings include absent voluntary external sphincter control, spastic bladder, and often uncoordinated activity of bladder and external sphincter. Chronically elevated intravesical pressure from DESD, if untreated, often leads to upper urinary tract deterioration. Classic urodynamic findings include uninhibited bladder contraction, simultaneous contraction of detrusor and external sphincter, high intravesical pressure, and high postvoid residual.

Lower urinary tract conditions associated with neurogenic bladder

Several secondary conditions occur as a result of LUT dysfunctions in spinal cord injuries. These conditions are caused by impaired LUT regulation, and their feared complications, if not treated appropriately, include upper urinary tract deterioration and eventual renal failure.

Detrusor (bladder) overactivity

Detrusor overactivity often occur in suprasacral spinal lesions in which the sacral reflex arc is intact; the end result is an overactive, uninhibited bladder caused by disruption of central (pontine) modulation of detrusor and external sphincter. Uninhibited bladder contraction during filling leads to high intravesical pressures that can be aggravated by the presence of DESD. In severe cases that are unresponsive to other therapeutic interventions, surgical defunctionalization of the detrusor can be considered, and can be in the form of either augmentation enterocystoplasty, bladder autoaugmentation, or conduit/continent diversions.

Bladder wall compliance

Another associated bladder dysfunction seen in neurogenic conditions is either an increase or decrease in bladder wall compliance; this is the ratio of a change in bladder volume to the associated change in intravesical pressure and is usually obtained from urodynamic study. A poorly compliant bladder distends with high intravesical pressure at relatively low volumes, and may lead to vesicoureteral reflux and places the upper urinary tract at even greater risk for deterioration [13–15]. A highly compliant bladder, conversely, is seen associated with a hyporeflexic or areflexic bladder as seen in lower motor neuron injuries. Intravesical pressures are generally low and, therefore, not harmful. Patients are usually unable to void and strict clean intermittent catheterization (CIC) is required to avoid overdistension injuries.

High leak-point detrusor pressure

The detrusor leak-point pressure (DLPP) is the maximum detrusor storage pressure at which leakage occurs from the bladder during passive filling and is determined from urodynamic studies. Sustained high detrusor pressure often results from a poorly compliant bladder and, when left uncorrected, further places the upper urinary tract at risk [16]. DLPP exceeding 40 cm H_2O is believed to place the upper tract at especially higher risk for deterioration [15,17].

Vesicoureteral reflux

Vesicoureteral reflux results from high DLPP and high intravesical pressure from low bladder compliance with or without detrusor-sphincter dyssynergia, and is associated with a higher risk for urinary tract infection [18] and upper tract deterioration [19]. Refluxing into the ureters and up to the kidneys leads to renal damage from pyelonephritis or ischemic injuries, with eventual renal scarring.

Detrusor-external sphincter dyssynergia

DESD is an intermittent or continuous involuntary contraction of the urethral sphincter during detrusor contraction. It is a common occurrence in suprasacral spinal cord lesions [20,21]. DESD has well-documented clinical significance, such as high detrusor pressure, vesicoureteral reflux, and upper tract deterioration [16,22]. Significant bladder outlet obstruction with associated high detrusor pressure may require transurethral sphincterotomy to reduce the detrusor pressure during voiding. Alternative treatment options, such as botulinum-A toxin injection into the external urethral sphincter, have also been used [23].

Investigational studies

Initial evaluation of the neurogenic bladder by a urologist in traumatic SCI usually occurs in the acute hospital setting once the patient is stable. This evaluation usually consists of an initial history, associated neurologic symptoms, and standard neurologic examination. Special attention must also be paid to sacral reflexes (ie, bulbocavernosal and cremasteric reflexes), sacral sensation, anal tone, and pelvic floor strength. Baseline testing should include urinalysis with microscopy and creatinine. In addition, upper urinary tract studies are useful for assessing baseline integrity. The upper urinary tract can be evaluated using renal ultrasound to assess for hydronephrosis, stones, and tumor, and kidney–ureter–bladder radiography to assess for renal or bladder stones. Other studies that can be performed as indicated or during long-term follow-up include voiding a cystogram, which assesses for vesicoureteral reflux, bladder hypertrophy, and bladder diverticula, and a dimercaptosuccinic acid renogram, which provides functional evaluation of the kidneys but offers less anatomic information. Cystoscopy is useful for direct visualization in cases of hematuria and persistent symptoms of irritation during voiding. It is used for long-term follow-up and helps identify bladder cancer and stones. A CT scan without a contrast-enhancing agent is another key imaging study and is the most sensitive means of evaluating for the presence of stones.

Urodynamic testing is the most definitive modality to assess dysfunction associated with neurogenic bladder; it helps in diagnosing the underlying voiding dysfunction and cause of LUT symptoms. Urodynamic testing is divided into a filling and storage/voiding phase. It combines multiple procedures, including cystometrogram, electromyography of the urethral sphincter, intra-abdominal pressure monitoring, and voiding cystourethrography. Information can be obtained on bladder filling and storage pressures, bladder compliance, and detrusor and sphincter activities. Baseline urodynamic testing is generally conducted once patients are stable, out of spinal shock, and performing intermittent catheterization. Information obtained from urodynamic studies are essential in guiding appropriate bladder management [24].

Continued urologic monitoring on a yearly basis or once every 2 years is required in patients who have spinal cord injuries. Routine follow-up urodynamic studies are required to assess changes in bladder pressures and current bladder dysfunction so that therapy can be altered as indicated [24]. The goal of continued follow-up is to preserve the upper urinary tract and prevent deterioration, although this may still occur despite an efficient bladder management program and LUT integrity [22].

Bladder management

Acute management

In the acute setting, patients who have SCI are usually in spinal shock with an associated areflexic, acontractile bladder and urinary retention generally lasting from 6 to 12 weeks; spinal shock, however, may last anywhere from a week to 12 months. The major goal in the acute setting is to preserve urinary tract integrity. Acute management of spinal cord injuries is generally achieved with an indwelling Foley catheter, which helps monitor urine output and is usually kept in place until patients are medically stable. Clean intermittent catheterization (CIC) can then be initiated. CIC is usually performed every 4 hours to maintain volumes at generally less than 500 mL; the schedule can be adjusted based on total fluid intake and urine volume output. Clean intermittent self-catheterization should be taught as early as possible to patients who have sufficient hand function. Patients should have a clear understanding of the need and goals of urologic management, which should ensure compliance.

Baseline blood urea nitrogen, creatinine, urinalysis, and urine culture and sensitivity are also usually obtained during acute hospitalization. Baseline urodynamic studies can be obtained, generally at approximately 6 weeks or as soon as urinary incontinence occurs. Urodynamics help guide appropriate bladder management. Ongoing routine urodynamic follow-up studies are then required to assess the need for adjustment in bladder management.

Optimum urologic management is also necessary for preventing autonomic dysreflexia in susceptible patients. Autonomic dysreflexia is an exaggerated sympathetic response to a noxious stimulus that occurs below the level of lesion in injuries at T6 or above. It is caused by lack of descending supraspinal inhibitory control and can be triggered by any bladder stimulus, such as overdistension, difficult catheterization, or even urodynamic studies.

Long-term management

The choice of long-term bladder management depends on many factors, including the level and completeness of injury, amount of hand function, sex, and motivation. Intermittent catheterization is now generally accepted as the best and safest long-term bladder management method [13]. The high rate of urologic complications that were once observed with chronic indwelling catheters are no longer as prevalent because of the routine use of CIC [25]. Chronic indwelling catheters (ie, Foley and suprapubic tubes) have often been shown to be associated with high rates of chronic urinary tract infections, urethritis, prostatitis, bladder stones, bladder diverticulae, strictures, abscesses, bladder cancer, and upper urinary tract disease such as pyelonephritis.

Lapides and colleagues [26] suggest that urinary tract infectious disease is based on overdistension of the bladder from urinary retention caused by ischemic changes in the bladder wall that then break down the tissue's defense mechanism against infection. Based on this theory, urinary retention, as opposed to catheterization per se, is the culprit for urinary tract infection. Intermittent catheterization would therefore prevent overdistension while flushing bacterial organisms from the bladder.

In patients who experience incontinence between catheterizations as a result of hyperreflexic bladder, pharmacologic interventions such as anticholinergic agents can be used.

Indwelling catheters: Foley catheter or suprapubic catheter

Long-term use of indwelling catheters, such as the Foley and suprapubic catheters, is no longer the primary means of bladder management;

intermittent catheterization has become the preferred method of bladder management secondary to less-associated complications [1,25,26]. In select patients, indwelling catheters may be used as less-invasive alternative forms of bladder management [27,28]. They are mainly used for patients who have limited hand functions to alleviate caregiver burden, and patients who have no motivation or refuse to perform other forms of bladder management. Complications from Foley catheters have been well documented, and include increased incidence of urinary tract infections; urethral diverticula; urethral strictures; urethritis; traumatic hypospadias; bladder calculi; small, low-compliance, high-pressure bladder; and bladder cancer [1,29–34].

Credé and Valsalva maneuvers

Injuries at the level of the conus or below (lower motor neuron injuries) result in an areflexic bladder with impaired detrusor contraction, large bladder capacity, and high residual urine. Bladder contraction and emptying in these instances can be facilitated with the Valsalva maneuver, which increases intra-abdominal pressure, or the Credé maneuver, which applies direct pressure to the suprapubic area.

Reflex voiding

In suprasacral lesions, the sacral reflex arc is generally intact with a resultant reflexic bladder. This physiology may allow reflex voiding using suprapubic tapping, which leads to bladder stimulation with subsequent contraction and opening of bladder neck. Reflex voiding is a much less popular method of bladder management and may be more suitable in male patients who lack adequate hand function for CIC, have longstanding SCI, and are able to drain the bladder to low postvoid residuals at scheduled intervals to avoid overdistension and urinary tract infections. However, because suprasacral lesions are often associated with detrusor-sphincter dyssynergia, elevated intravesical voiding pressures may be associated, with resultant deleterious effects on the upper urinary tract. This method of voiding is generally used with an external collecting device and often requires transurethral sphincterotomy to allow bladder drainage at low pressure.

Pharmacologic management

Systemic medications

The goal of most pharmacologic agents used for treating neurogenic bladder associated with SCI has been to inhibit involuntary detrusor activity and, as a result, increase bladder capacity and reduce intravesical pressures. The main classes of pharmacologic agents currently used are anticholinergics (eg, oxybutynin, tolterodine), tricyclic antidepressants (eg, imipramine, which has strong antimuscarinic actions), and antispasmodic drugs (eg, baclofen, tizanidine). The use of anticholinergic medications, however, may be associated with significant undesirable effects, such as dry mouth and impaired gastrointestinal secretion and motility. Oxybutynin can also be administered intravesically, although systemic absorption does occur.

Intravesical therapy

The injection of botulinum toxin type A (BTX-A) into the detrusor muscle as a nonsurgical treatment alternative for neurogenic detrusor activity was initially introduced by Schurch and colleagues [35]. BTX-A is the most widely used serotype for therapeutic purposes. Botulinum toxin has a high affinity for cholinergic peripheral nerve endings and inhibits acetylcholine release at neuromuscular junctions, resulting in prolonged local muscular weakness and paralysis when injected directly into muscle [36]. This effect is reversible, with a reported length of action on the detrusor muscle between 16 and 36 weeks [12,35,37,38]. Undesirable side effects associated with local injection of BTX-A are not generally seen compared with other pharmacologic interventions, such as anticholinergics [35,38], which is likely the result of no toxin spilling into the circulatory system from tight binding at local intramuscular nerve terminals [36].

For detrusor overactivity, the toxin is injected in the detrusor muscle into multiple sites at a dose generally between 200 and 300 units [35,38]; higher doses may be associated with an increased risk for developing antibodies to the toxin, with possible associated treatment failure [39]. The ultimate effect of injecting the detrusor with botulinum toxin is suppression of bladder overactivity, increase in cystometric and maximum bladder capacity, decrease in voiding pressure, and elimination of urinary incontinence that may be associated with detrusor overactivity [35,38]. This intravesical treatment option for neurogenic detrusor overactivity seems to be a safe and suitable nonsurgical alternative for patients who have severe neurogenic incontinence, especially if they are unresponsive to other pharmacologic agents, such as anticholinergics. Patients who have underlying low compliance may not experience any benefit from BTX-A injection, because of possible detrusor muscle changes such as fibrosis [35]. BTX-A injection into the external urethral sphincter is also used to treat neurogenic detrusor-sphincter dyssynergia and improves voiding [23]. The major drawback of BTX-A is the temporary effect, necessitating repeat injections approximately every 6 months.

Other intravesical therapies to treat detrusor overactivity have been tried. These act through different mechanisms and may reduce or eliminate some of the systemic side effects seen with oral medication. These therapeutic options have included intravesical injections of oxybutynin, atropine, local anesthetics, vallinoids, resiniferatoxin, nociceptin/orphanin FQ, and capsaicin [40].

Surgical management

Electrical stimulation and posterior sacral root rhizotomy

In spinal cord injuries from suprasacral lesions, electrical stimulation of sacral anterior nerve roots has been used to produce effective micturition with relatively low residual volumes. Electrodes are surgically implanted on sacral nerves with the stimulator placed under the skin, generally the abdomen. Stimulation is provided directly to the S3 nerve root and suppresses hyperreflexic detrusor activity. This mechanism is often combined with division of the posterior sacral roots and is intended to eliminate detrusor and sphincter hyperreflexia, increase bladder capacity and compliance, and decrease incidence of reflex incontinence.

Augmentation cystoplasty, cutaneous conduits, and urinary diversions

Various other forms of surgical continence measures are available when primary bladder management methods fail. These include augmentation cystoplasty and various cutaneous conduits/urinary diversion methods wherein the ureters are connected to an intestinal segment that is externalized through the abdominal wall, draining into an external collecting device. Urinary diversions are sometimes performed in women who have difficulty performing catheterization and patients who have complications caused by indwelling catheters, perineal decubiti, and bladder malignancy requiring cystectomy.

The goal of bladder augmentation (or augmentation enterocystoplasty) is to increase total bladder capacity. In patients who have SCI with neurogenic bladder dysfunction refractory to conservative management, this procedure is intended to increase detrusor compliance and lower bladder storage pressures that may place the upper tracts at risk for deterioration [42]. The basic procedure involves using a bowel segment, such as the ileum, right colon, descending/sigmoid colon, or stomach, to augment the bladder (Fig. 4). It

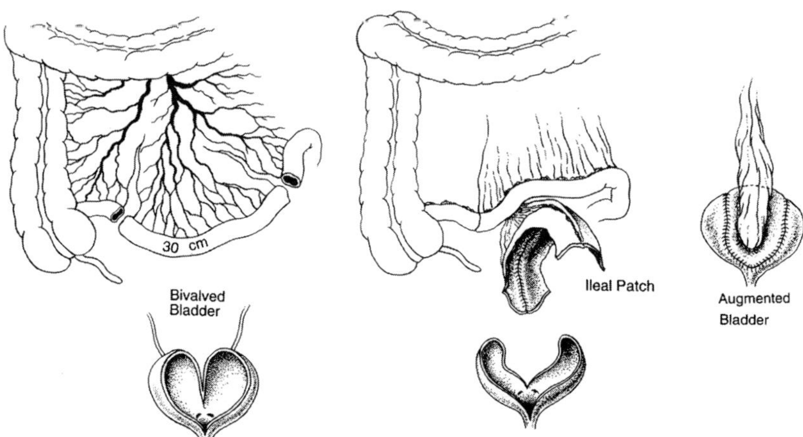

Fig. 4. Augmentation cystoplasty. A 30-cm segment of small bowel is opened and reconstructed as s U-shaped patch and then sewn into the bivalved bladder. (*From* Cardenas DD, Mayo ME, King JC. Urinary tract and bowel management in the rehabilitation setting. In: Braddom RL, Buschbacher RM, Dumitru D, et al, editors. Physical medicine and rehabilitation. Philadelphia: W.B. Saunders; 1996. p. 555–79; with permission.)

is an irreversible procedure and should be used for patients who have undergone failed conservative medical management in the setting of high detrusor pressures. An alternative surgical approach is detrusor myomectomy through excision of the submucosa, creating a weakened muscle and resultant diverticulum [43]. An alternative surgical approach is detrusor myomectomy through excision of the submucosa, creating a weakened muscle and resultant diverticulum [43]. In most cases, spontaneous voiding after surgery will likely not occur, and permanent intermittent catheterization is the norm. Long-term complications, most notably metabolic derangements and change in bowel habits, depend on the segment of bowel used.

Diverting the urine from the LUT and perineum might become necessary for some patients who have SCI who have difficulties with catheterization, have urethral or penile skin changes such as fistulae or strictures, or experience incontinence that impairs management of decubitus ulcers [44]. Supravesical conduits or continent diversions using a bowel segment are performed when a bladder neck closure or suprapubic tube placement is not an option [44]. The simplest surgical method is the ileal conduit. In this method, an adequate length of bowel segment is resected, the ureters are implanted at the proximal end of this segment, and the distal end is externalized through the abdominal wall. Subsequent urostomy care is performed with relative ease as opposed to a continent stoma. This conduit is not a urine storage reservoir; there is only transient contact of urine with the absorptive surface, and therefore no significant metabolic derangement is seen compared with other forms of surgical bladder management. Continued routine monitoring of basic metabolic profile, renal function, and the upper tracts for deterioration is required.

Continent urinary diversions can be of two forms: one in which the reservoir is attached to the urethra as opposed to the bladder (orthotopic diversions) or one that can be catheterized through an abdominal stoma. The latter can provide easy accessibility to patients who have SCI, because little effort is required to insert the catheter through the stoma. This method is ideal for paraplegics who have cystectomies or significant decubitus ulcers and for paraplegic female patients who have technically difficult catheterizations. However, it may not be beneficial for high-tetraplegic patients who may lack the ability to perform self-catheterization and for patients unlikely to be compliant with appropriate care instructions [44]. This surgical method involves the resection of a lengthy segment of small and large bowel (usually for terminal ileum to the ascending colon past the hepatic flexure) as reservoir system. This segment of bowel is sewn into a closed pouch to which the ureters are attached, and the terminal ileum is then externalized through the abdominal wall; the ileocecal valve provides a continence mechanism. This structure is a storage mechanism that allows prolonged contact of urine with the absorptive surface of bowel and can be associated with significant metabolic derangements. Therefore, careful patient selection and follow-up is mandatory.

Transurethral sphincterotomy

Transurethral sphincterotomy is the transurethral surgical incision of the external urinary sphincter in cases of bladder outlet obstruction secondary to DESD, allowing subsequent use of an external collecting device. This procedure has been mainstay of treatment for significant DESD with associated elevated detrusor voiding pressure unresponsive to anticholinergic agents. The decrease in outlet resistance theoretically lowers the high detrusor pressures associated with DESD and averts the need for an indwelling catheter. It is typically performed in male quadriplegic or high-thoracic paraplegic patients who have difficulties performing CIC secondary to poor hand function.

Complications of neurogenic bladder

Urologic complications that have been associated with neurogenic bladder, although less prevalent with the widespread use of CIC, are still a major concern. Many such urologic complications still exist, however, and amongst those are chronic urinary tract infections, bladder diverticulae, bladder stones, urethral trauma leading to penile fistulae or strictures, perineal decubiti, bladder cancer, vesicoureteral reflux, hydronephrosis, pyelonephritis, and renal failure.

Persistent bacteriuria is not uncommon in patients who have SCI and asymptomatic bacteriuria is often found regardless of the type of bladder management, including indwelling catheters, intermittent catheterization, or external collecting devices. Patients who have SCI become particularly at high risk to urinary tract infections secondary to bladder overdistension from urinary retention, vesicoureteral reflux, high detrusor pressures, chronic stone disease, and various forms of resultant bladder outlet obstruction, such as detrusor-sphincter dyssynergia, strictures, and instrumentation. Treatment of asymptomatic bacteriuria or prophylactic use of antibiotics is not usually recommended [45–49]. Routine cultures are not generally required and symptoms such as fever, sweating, chills, nausea and vomiting, gross pyuria, increased spasticity, and abdominal or costovertebral tenderness must be present for treatment to be initiated. In cases of urease-producing pathogens (eg, *Proteus, Pseudomonas, Klebsiella*) or in the presence of reflux, however, treatment of asymptomatic bacteriuria is often recommended [50].

The SCI population has a high incidence of renal stone disease, especially in the presence of vesicoureteral reflux [31,51]. Infection with urea-splitting bacteria is a significant predisposing factor for formation of these stones, and the prophylactic use of acetohydroxamic acid can help reduce the incidence of these stones [41]. Other associated risk factors in renal stone formation include hypercalcemia, older age, complete neurologic injury, previous history of bladder calculi, sepsis, and indwelling catheters [53–55].

An important complication of neurogenic bladder caused by SCI is vesicoureteral reflux and upper tract deterioration. Upper tract deterioration is often the result of low detrusor compliance and high detrusor pressures, which lead to vesicoureteral reflux with or without hydronephrosis [13–15,56]. Some studies report that the incidence of vesicoureteral reflux and hydronephrosis with associated low bladder compliance and elevated intravesical pressures in the SCI population is high [14,15]. In the presence of bacteriuria, the upper tract becomes at even greater risk for infection, stones, and, ultimately, deterioration [57]. Vesicoureteral reflux is generally managed conservatively with anticholinergic agents and CIC, except in the case of persistent high-grade reflux in which case ureteral reimplantation might be indicated.

Bladder cancer, although rare, is another important complication associated with neurogenic bladder, mostly associated with chronic indwelling catheters [58]. Squamous cell carcinoma is the most common histologic type, which may or may not be seen in association with elements of transitional cell carcinoma [58–61]. The incidence of bladder carcinoma in patients who have SCI has been reported to be between 2% and 10% [52,59,60]. The use of chronic indwelling catheters has been identified as an important risk factor, with the risk related proportionately to the duration of chronic indwelling catheter use [52,59,62], and may be related to chronic irritation and infection of the urothelium, leading to urothelial dysplastic changes and squamous metaplasia [63]. Although squamous metaplasia is often seen in patients who have SCI and a chronic indwelling catheter, whether it directly progresses to cancer is unclear [59]. Typical symptoms associated with bladder cancer are gross or microscopic hematuria or recurrent urinary tract infections [59,60]. Cystoscopy is the preferred diagnostic study, often revealing the underlying pathology; it should be routine in patients who have longstanding indwelling catheters, along with upper urinary tract evaluation [59]. Squamous cell cancer of the bladder is a rather aggressive tumor, which is often metastatic at diagnosis. The prognosis is poor and radical cystectomy is the preferred treatment.

Special considerations

Women

Because women account for only 20% of all patients who have SCI, specific studies addressing their unique concerns are few. As in men, intermittent catheterization is the preferred method for bladder emptying in those who have adequate hand function or adequate caregiver assistance to perform the catheterization [64]. Women in general, however, experience more technical difficulties with intermittent urethral catheterization than men, especially in tetraplegia [65]. Another main difference is the unavailability of any suitable external incontinence device (ie, the male counterpart of a condom catheter). These issues have often led to the use of indwelling catheters as the primary mode of bladder management in women. The use of long-term indwelling catheters is often associated with labial and urethral erosion and resultant leakage around the catheter, with associated skin conditions [64,66]. Elevated intravesical pressures and prevention of leakage can be managed in some instances with the addition of anticholinergics to intermittent catheterization [66]. When intermittent catheterization is not a suitable option, such as in severe incontinence and urine leakage around the catheter, augmentation cystoplasty or some form of urinary diversion or cutaneous continent conduit should be considered. Transurethral sphincterotomy is generally not a consideration in women because of the lack of a suitable external incontinence device.

Pediatric patients

Children represent a small portion of the SCI population. In numerous instances, the injuries are congenital from myelodysplasia. Management of neurogenic bladder must consider the child's normal developmental process, psychomotor skills, and any cognitive limitations that may be the result of age or brain injury. Intermittent catheterization remains the preferred bladder management method and, as much as possible, the child's participation should be encouraged. When appropriate, children should be allowed to perform their own self-catheterization. In uninhibited bladder from upper motor neuron injuries, timed voiding may be effective in maintaining continence. The use of latex-free catheters and gloves are generally recommended, especially in spina bifida, because of latex allergies. With acquired injuries, toileting must be relearned and comfort with toileting devices acquired.

References

[1] Donnelly J, Hackler RH, Bunts RC. Present urologic status of the World War II paraplegic: 25-year followup. Comparison with status of the 20-year Korean War paraplegic and 5-year Vietnam paraplegic. J Urol 1972;108:558–62.

[2] Borges PM, Hackler RH. The urologic status of the Vietnam War paraplegic: a 15-year prospective followup. J Urol 1982;127:710–1.

[3] Hackler RH. A 25-year prospective mortality study in the spinal cord-injured patient: comparison with long-term living paraplegic. J Urol 1977;117:486–8.

[4] Matsui M, Motomura D, Fujikawa T, et al. Mice lacking M2 and M3 muscarinic acetylcholine receptors are devoid of cholinergic smooth muscle contractions but still viable. J Neurosci 2002;22:10627–32.

[5] Andersson KE, Arner A. Urinary bladder contraction and relaxation: physiology and pathophysiology. Physiol Rev 2004;84:935–86.

[6] Habler HJ, Janig W, Koltzenburg M. Activation of unmyelinated afferent fibres by mechanical stimuli and inflammation of the urinary bladder in the cat. J Physiol 1990;425:545–62.

[7] Thor K, Morgan C, Nadelhaft I, et al. Organization of afferent and efferent pathways in the pudendal nerve of the female cat. J Comp Neurol 1989;288:263–79.

[8] DeGroat WC, Theobald RJ. Reflex activation of sympathetic pathways to vesical smooth muscle and parasympathetic ganglia by electrical stimulation of vesical afferents. J Phys 1976;259:223–37.

[9] Mallory BS, Roppolo JR, De Groat WC. Pharmacological modulation of the pontine micturition center. Brain Res 1991;546:310–20.

[10] DeGroat WC. Nervous control of the urinary bladder of the cat. Brain Res 1975;87:201–11.
[11] Bors E, Comarr AE. Neurological urology; physiology of micturition, its neurological disorders and sequelae. Baltimore (MD): University Park Press; 1971.
[12] Leippold T, Reitz A, Schurch B. Botulinum toxin as a new therapy option for voiding disorders: current state of the art. Eur Urol 2003;44:165–74.
[13] Weld KJ, Graney MJ, Dmochowski RR. Differences in bladder compliance with time and association of bladder management with compliance in spinal cord injured patients. J Urol 2000;163:1228–33.
[14] Hackler RH, Hall MK, Zampieri TA. Bladder hypocompliance in the spinal cord injury population. J Urol 1989;141(6):1390–3.
[15] McGuire EJ, Woodside JR, Borden TA, et al. Prognostic value of urodynamic testing in myelodysplastic patients. J Urol 1981;126:205–9.
[16] Gerridzen RG, Thijssen AM, Dehoux E. Risk factors for upper tract deterioration in chronic spinal cord injury patients. J Urol 1992;147:416–8.
[17] Bennett CJ, Young M, Parrington H. Leak point pressure assessment of new spinal cord injury patients. Chicago: American Spinal Injury Association; 1990.
[18] De Ruz AE, Leoni EG, Cabrera RH. Epidemiology and risk factors for urinary tract infection in patients with spinal cord injury. J Urol 2000;164:1285–9.
[19] Ku JH, Choi WJ, Lee KY, et al. Complications of the upper urinary tract in patients with spinal cord injury: a long-term follow-up study. Urol Res 2005;33:435–9.
[20] Weld KJ, Dmochowski RR. Association of level of injury and bladder behavior in patients with post-traumatic spinal cord injury. Urology 2000;55:490–4.
[21] Kaplan SA, Chancellor MB, Blaivas JG. Bladder and sphincter behaviors in patients with spinal cord lesions. J Urol 1991;146:113–7.
[22] Perkash I. Detrusor-sphincter dyssynergia and detrusor hyperreflexia leading to hydronephrosis during intermittent catheterization. J Urol 1978;120:620–2.
[23] Schurch B, Hauri D, Rodic B, et al. Botulinum-A toxin as a treatment of detrusor-sphincter dyssynergia: a prospective study in 24 spinal cord injury patients. J Urol 1996;155:1023–9.
[24] Abrams P, Cardoza L, Fall M, et al. The standardization of terminology in lower urinary tract function: report from the standardization sub-committee of International Continence Society. Urology 2003;61:37–49.
[25] Weld KJ, Dmochowski RR. Effect of bladder management on urological complications in spinal cord injured patients. J Urol 2000;163:768–72.
[26] Lapides J, Diokno AC, Silber SM, et al. Clean, intermittent self-catheterization in the treatment of urinary tract disease. 1972. J Urol 2002;167:1584–6.
[27] Dewire DM, Owens RS, Anderson GA, et al. A comparison of the urological complications associated with long-term management of quadriplegics with and without chronic indwelling urinary catheters. J Urol 1992;147:1069–71.
[28] MacDiarmid SA, Arnold EP, Palmer NB, et al. Management of spinal cord injured patients by indwelling suprapubic catheterization. J Urol 1995;154:492–4.
[29] Weld KJ, Wall BM, Mangold TA, et al. Influences on renal function in chronic spinal cord injured patients. J Urol 2000;164(5):1490–3.
[30] Kuhn W, Rist M, Zaech GA. Intermittent urethral self-catheterization: long-term results. Paraplegia 1991;29:222–32.
[31] Hall MK, Hackler RH, Zampieri TA, et al. Renal calculi in spinal cord-injured patients: association with reflux, bladder stones, and Foley catheter drainage. Urology 1989;34:126–8.
[32] Hardy AG. Complications of the indwelling catheter. Paraplegia 1968;6:5–10.
[33] Warren JW, Tenney JH, Hoopes JM, et al. A prospective microbiologic study of bacteriuria in patients with chronic indwelling urethral catheters. J Infect Dis 1982;146:719–23.
[34] Kyle EW. The complications of indwelling catheters. Paraplegia 1968;6:1–4.
[35] Schurch B, Stöhrer M, Kramer G, et al. Botulinum-A toxin for treating detrusor hyperreflexia in spinal cord injury patients: a new alternative to anticholinergic drugs? Preliminary results. J Urol 2000;164:692–7.

[36] Simpson LL. The origin, structure and pharmacological activity of botulinum toxin. Pharmacol Rev 1981;33:155–88.
[37] Reitz A, Stöhre M, Kramer G, et al. European experience of 200 cases treated with botulinum-A toxin injections into the detrusor muscle for urinary incontinence due to neurogenic detrusor overactivity. Eur Urol 2004;45:510–5.
[38] Klaphajone J, Kitisomprayoonkul W, Sriplakit S. Botulinum toxin type A injections for the treatment of neurogenic detrusor overactivity combined with low-compliance bladder in patients with spinal cord lesions. Arch Phys Med Rehabil 2005;86:2114–8.
[39] Clinical use of Botulinum toxin. National Institute of Health Consensus Development Conference Statement, Nov 12-14. Arch Neurol 1991;48:1294–8.
[40] Reitz A, Schurch B. Intravesical therapy options for neurogenic detrusor overactivity. Spinal Cord 2004;42:267–72.
[41] Griffith DP, Khonsari F, Skurnick JH, et al. A randomized trial of acetohydroxamic acid for the treatment and prevention of infection-induced urinary stones in spinal cord injury patients. J Urol 1988;140(2):318–24.
[42] Queek ML, Ginsberg DA. Long-term urodynamics followup of bladder augmentation for neurogenic bladder. J Urol 2003;169:195–8.
[43] Appell RA. Surgery for the treatment on overactive bladder. Urology 1998;51:27–9.
[44] Razi SS, Bennett CJ. Selecting the appropriate urinary diversion procedure in the spinal cord injured: a poignant reminder. J Spinal Cord Med 1996;19:197–200.
[45] Infectious Diseases Society of America guidelines for the diagnosis and treatment of asymptomatic bacteriuria in adults. Clin Infect Dis 2005;40:643–54.
[46] Breitenbucher RB. Bacterial changes in the urine samples of patients with long term indwelling catheters. Arch Intern Med 1984;144:1585–8.
[47] Maynard FM, Diokno AC. Urinary infection and complications during clean intermittent catheterization following spinal cord injury. J Urol 1984;132:943–6.
[48] Erickson RP, Merritt JL, Opitz JL, et al. Bacteriuria during follow-up in patients with spinal cord injury: I. Rates of bacteriuria in various bladder-emptying methods. Arch Phys Med Rehabil 1982;63:409–12.
[49] Mohler JL, Cowen DL, Flanigan RC. Suppression and treatment of urinary tract infection in patients with an intermittently catheterized neurogenic bladder. J Urol 1987; 138:336–40.
[50] Maynard F, Cardenas D, Krause J, et al. National Institute on Disability and Rehabilitation. The prevention and management of urinary infections among people with spinal injuries. J Am Paraplegia Soc 1992;15:194–204.
[51] DeVivo MJ, Fine PR, Cutter GR, et al. The risk of renal calculi in spinal cord injury patients. J Urol 1984;131:857–60.
[52] Locke JR, Hill DE, Walzer Y. Incidence of squamous cell carcinoma in patients with long-term catheter drainage. J Urol 1985;133:1034–5.
[53] Ku JH, Jung TY, Lee JK, et al. Risk factors for urinary stone formation in men with spinal cord injury: a 17-year follow-up study. BJU Int 2006;97:790–3.
[54] Chen Y, DeVivo MJ, Roseman JM. Current trend and risk factors for kidney stones in persons with spinal cord injury: a longitudinal study. Spinal Cord 2000;38:346–53.
[55] Ord J, Lunn D, Reynard J. Bladder management and risk of bladder stone formation in spinal cord injured patients. J Urol 2003;170:1734–7.
[56] Yokoyama O, Hasegawa T, Ishiura Y, et al. Morphological and functional factors predicting bladder deterioration after spinal cord injury. J Urol 1996;155:271–4.
[57] Hackler RH, Katz PG. Management of common problems in spinal cord injured patients. Am Urol Assoc Update Ser (Vol. X, lesson 6) 1991;10:42–7.
[58] West DA, Cummings JM, Longo WE, et al. Role of chronic catheterization in the development of bladder cancer in patients with spinal cord injury. Urology 1999;53:292–7.
[59] Kaufmann JM, Fam B, Jacobs SC, et al. Bladder cancer and squamous metaplasia in spinal cord injury patients. J Urol 1977;118:967–71.

[60] Bejany DE, Lockhart JL, Rhamy RK. Malignant vesical tumors following spinal cord injury. J Urol 1987;138:1390–2.
[61] Bickel A, Culkin DJ, Wheeler JS. Bladder cancer in spinal cord injury patients. J Urol 1991; 146:1240–2.
[62] Stonehill WH, Dmochowski RR, Patterson AL, et al. Risk factors for bladder tumors in spinal cord injury patients. J Urol 1996;155:1248–52.
[63] Goble NM, Clarke TJ, Hammonds JC. Histological changes in the urinary bladder secondary to urethral catheterization. Br J Urol 1989;63:354–7.
[64] McGuire EJ, Savastano JA. Comparative urologic outcome in women with spinal cord injury. J Urol 1986;135:730–1.
[65] Lindan R, Leffler EJ, Bodner D. Urologic problems in the management of quadriplegic women. Paraplegia 1987;25:381–5.
[66] Bennett CJ, Young MN, Adkins RH, et al. Comparison of the bladder management complication outcomes in female spinal cord injury patients. J Urol 1995;153:1458–60.

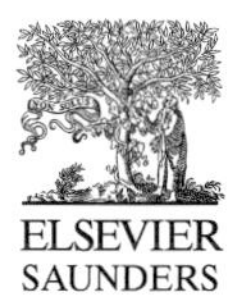

ELSEVIER
SAUNDERS

Phys Med Rehabil Clin N Am
18 (2007) 275–296

PHYSICAL MEDICINE
AND REHABILITATION
CLINICS OF
NORTH AMERICA

Autonomic Nervous System Dysfunction After Spinal Cord Injury

Susan V. Garstang, MD*, Stacey A. Miller-Smith, MD

Department of Physical Medicine and Rehabilitation, UMNDJ-New Jersey Medical School, 30 Bergen Street, ADMC 101, Newark, NJ 07039, USA

The intact spinal cord is responsible for carrying and modulating many types of signals, both those of the somatic nervous system, which is involved in motor and sensory processes, but also the myriad of functions occurring under the control of the autonomic nervous system (ANS). After spinal cord injury (SCI), damage to the autonomic pathways that travel in the spinal cord leads to altered regulation of many processes that are subsumed by the autonomic nervous system. The ANS regulates many functions, including control of cardiovascular functions such as coronary blood flow, cardiac contractility, heart rate, and peripheral vasomotor responses. In addition, the autonomic nervous system controls blood flow to skeletal muscle, kidneys, the splanchnic circulation, and the skin. Impaired ANS regulation caused by SCI leads to many of the clinical issues seen in persons with SCI, including altered cardiovascular and thermoregulatory function and manifestations of end-organ dysfunction, such as neurogenic bowel and bladder. This review focuses mainly on the effects of autonomic nervous system dysfunction on cardiovascular control in individuals with SCI.

Elements of autonomic nervous system dysfunction after SCI can be divided into acute and chronic processes, with some overlap. Acutely, neurogenic shock occurs with its component hypotension, hypothermia, and bradycardia. Hypotension and bradycardia last 2 to 6 weeks and are accompanied by arrhythmias that occur primarily in the acute setting. Pulmonary effects of disruption of sympathetic innervation in persons with tetraplegia also are of importance in the period immediately after injury. Orthostatic hypotension occurs acutely but is clinically more relevant during the postacute phase during rehabilitation when mobilization is occurring. However, some patients have long-term orthostasis. Chronic manifestations of

* Corresponding author.
E-mail address: garstasv@umdnj.edu (S.V. Garstang).

doi:10.1016/j.pmr.2007.02.003 **pmr.theclinics.com**

autonomic dysfunction include impaired temperature regulation and impaired cardiovascular function and responses to exercise. Autonomic dysreflexia is also caused by altered autonomic nervous system function but will not be covered in this review.

Autonomic nervous system anatomy

The ANS has two components or divisions that may be disrupted as a result of damage to the spinal cord, the parasympathetic nervous system (PNS) and the sympathetic nervous system (SNS). The enteric nervous system, also considered a division of the ANS, is not directly disrupted after SCI. The level and extent of injury to the spinal cord determines the dysfunction that occurs. A thorough understanding of the anatomy is important in predicting the types of alterations in function that will occur after spinal cord injury.

The autonomic nervous system controls many functions via complex pathways, typically with the sympathetic division and parasympathetic division serving opposing regulatory roles. These reflex pathways consist of sensory receptors, afferent pathways, integration centers in the central nervous system (CNS), efferent pathways, and effector organs [1]. Ascending and descending impulses are generally carried in the spinal cord (with the exception of the cranial parasympathetic division) and connect with interneurons, which begin in the CNS, traverse the ventral roots, and terminate in an ANS ganglion outside the CNS. These interneurons are called *preganglionic neurons*, and the effector neurons that originate in the ANS ganglion are called postganglionic neurons [2]. Both divisions of the autonomic nervous system have preganglionic and postganglionic neurons. The cell bodies of the preganglionic neurons lie in the brain or spinal cord. The cell bodies of the postganglionic neuron lie in autonomic ganglia, which are located either near the spinal cord or near the effector organ. The viscera are innervated by both divisions of the ANS, which typically provide opposing regulatory controls. However, some blood vessels and sweat glands have only a single type of innervation.

The PNS has cell bodies in the brainstem and sacral spinal cord and thus is often referred to as the *craniosacral division of the ANS*. The preganglionic fibers arise in the visceral brainstem nuclei and the second through fourth sacral segments. The cranial nerve fibers are carried with cranial nerves III, VII, IX, and X and innervate structures in the head and neck as well as thoracic and abdominal viscera. The preganglionic parasympathetic fibers that innervate the descending colon and pelvic organs originate in the sacral segments. The spinal cord has the important role of carrying efferent impulses from the brainstem via the lateral reticulospinal tract to the sacral cord. Most preganglionic parasympathetic fibers synapse in the inferior mesenteric ganglion, but some continue without synapsing through the hypogastric nerves to reach the vesical plexus in the bladder wall [3].

The SNS has cell bodies in the intermediolateral or intermediomedial cell columns of the spinal cord, and the preganglionic fibers leave the cord and join the ventral roots of T1 to L2. Hence, this division is often referred to as the *thoracolumbar division*. Variations in level of origin do occur, and preganglionic fibers from as high as C7 to as low as L4 have been shown [3]. Preganglionic fibers typically run in the spinal cord for several levels, and in fact some remain intraspinal for up to 12 levels. In addition, some of the fibers cross while others remain uncrossed. In general, axons destined for thoracic ganglia tend to be unilateral, whereas those going to lumber ganglia are typically bilateral.

Preganglionic sympathetic fibers may synapse in the paravertebral ganglia of the sympathetic chain located on either side of the vertebral bodies or in collateral (prevertebral) ganglia located near the viscera [3]. Above the diaphragm, all sympathetic preganglionic fibers synapse in the sympathetic chain. In the cervical region, there are several paravertebral ganglia, namely the superior cervical ganglion, the middle cervical ganglion, and the stellate ganglion (consists of the inferior cervical ganglion and first thoracic ganglion) [2]. In the thoracic region there are up to 11 paravertebral ganglia. There are four lumbar and four sacral paravertebral ganglia. The chain ganglia in the coccygeal region are fused into the coccygeal ganglion or ganglion impar.

Preganglionic sympathetic fibers to the abdominal and pelvic viscera travel through the paravertebral ganglia without synapsing and then form splanchnic nerves. These fibers synapse with the postganglionic neurons, which are located in collateral ganglia, and the fibers then travel with major arteries to the effector organs. The superior and infection mesenteric ganglia are examples of collateral ganglia in which pre- and postganglionic fibers synapse. The postganglionic fibers of the SNS also form visceral nerves, such as the cardiac nerves, and join peripheral nerves to innervate blood vessels and the skin.

The heart is innervated by both sympathetic and parasympathetic postganglionic fibers. Cardiac sympathetic preganglionic neurons synapse with postganglionic neurons in the middle cervical ganglia and stellate ganglion [4]. Cardiac parasympathetic fibers originate in the dorsal motor nucleus of the vagus and the nucleus ambiguous in the medulla oblongata and travel in the recurrent laryngeal nerves and vagus nerve [5]. These nerves interconnect with sympathetic cardiopulmonary nerves near the pulmonary artery to form the ventral and dorsal cardiopulmonary plexuses [6]. Emerging from these plexuses are three large cardiac nerves as well as several small cardiac nerves, which serve to innervate the conduction system, the atria, and the ventricles. Parasympathetic fibers synapse with postganglionic cells on the epicardial surface or within the walls of the heart near the sinoatrial (SA) or atrioventricular (AV) node.

Autonomic nervous system physiology

The autonomic nervous system regulates all essential physiologic components of circulation including heart rate, stroke volume, and vascular resistance, which, in turn, determine arterial blood pressure and cardiac output.

The autonomic nervous system regulates these functions in response to feedback from afferent pathways by affecting the force and frequency of cardiac contraction and vasodilation or vasoconstriction. Other influences have a role in the final physiologic state, including hormonal and local metabolic factors and intravascular volume.

Control of cardiovascular function is via a complex system of feedback loops that modulate sympathetic and parasympathetic input. Arterial chemoreceptors, ergoreceptors in skeletal muscle, and cardiopulmonary receptors with sympathetic afferents provide excitatory input to the nucleus tractus solitarius [2]. Parasympathetic afferents transmit information from the aortic arch and carotid baroreceptors as well as receptors in the systemic and pulmonary vessels, the great veins, and the atria. These afferent impulses travel in cranial nerve IX (glossopharyngeal) and X (vagus) to provide inhibitory input to the nucleus tractus solitarius [7].

The arterial baroreceptors located in the aortic arch and carotid sinuses respond to a reduction in arterial pressure by decreasing activity of the parasympathetic nerves and increasing activity of the sympathetic excitatory nerves. In contrast, the baroreceptors respond to an increase in arterial pressure by stimulation of the spinal sympathetic inhibitory tract, inhibition of the spinal sympathetic excitatory tract, and stimulation of the activity of parasympathetic preganglionic nerves [1]. Via these feedback controls, the sympathetic outflow is modulated, with parasympathetic outflow serving an inhibitory role.

Heart rate and rhythmicity are also under the control of the autonomic nervous system. The SA node is under direct influence of both the SNS and PNS. Sympathetic input increases the rate at which the SA node generates action potentials, and parasympathetic input decreases the rate of action potential generation [8].

The SNS exerts primary control of blood flow to the skin, kidneys, and splanchnic organs, whereas local metabolic influences exert primary control over blood flow to the heart and skeletal muscle [9]. The splanchnic circulation supplies blood flow to the abdominal organs, including the gastrointestinal tract, spleen, pancreas, and liver. These organs receive about 25% of resting cardiac output and contain more than 20% of circulating blood volume. The arteries and veins of these organs are richly innervated with sympathetic vasoconstrictor nerves, thus, activation of the SNS can produce an 80% reduction in flow in the splanchnic circulation and cause a large shift of blood to the central circulation [9]. Renal blood flow also decreases during SNS activation, and low perfusion pressures are thought to trigger the release of renin.

The final outcome of all these processes is regulation of systemic vascular resistance and cardiac filling pressure (and thus stroke volume and cardiac output), which, in turn, control arterial blood pressure. Table 1 delineates the sympathetic outflow by effector organ, receptor, neurotransmitter type, and function (data from Ref. [2]).

Table 1
Overview of sympathetic outflow to target organs

Target organ or structure	Heart: coronary arteries, sinus node, conduction system	Kidney: juxtaglomerular cells	Systemic resistance vessels	Capacitance vessels: primarily splanchnic	Adrenal medulla
Adrenoreceptor type	Beta	Beta	Beta	Beta	Alpha
Neurotransmitter	NA	NA	NA	NA	ACh
Function	Regulates heart rate, cardiac contractility, coronary blood flow	Release of renin	Vasoconstriction: Regulates SVR	Vasoconstriction: Regulates cardiac filling pressure and stroke volume	Release of circulating adrenaline, which also activates vascular β-receptors.

Abbreviations: ACh, acetylcholine; NA, noradrenaline; SVR, systemic vascular resistance.

Autonomic nervous system control of thermoregulation

Thermoregulatory responses depend on cold and warm sensors in the hypothalamus and the skin but also on input from mesencephalic, medullary, spinal, and intra-abdominal temperature sensors [2,10]. Afferent fibers from the peripheral receptors with cell bodies in the dorsal root ganglia enter the spinal cord and ascend contralaterally to the medial lemniscus and the thalamus and then project further to the hypothalamus [2,11]. The preoptic area of the hypothalamus controls the thermal set-point and integrates thermoregulatory responses [2,11]. The efferents from the hypothalamus control thermoregulatory vasomotor and sudomotor tone as well as nonshivering and shivering thermogenesis via descending noradrenergic and cholinergic fibers that exit the spinal cord below C-7 [2,11].

Sympathetic nervous system control of the skin contributes to thermoregulation. At rest, the skin receives 6% of resting cardiac output. This can be reduced markedly if heat needs to be retained and increase up to seven times normal if heat needs to be dissipated. A reduction in sympathetic vasoconstrictor tone causes vasodilation, because the venous plexus in the skin is richly innervated with sympathetic vasoconstrictor nerves [9].

When the body is exposed to temperatures greater than 30°C, there is progressive cutaneous vasodilation, which enhances heat loss to the environment [2]. Heat loss by evaporation provides the major physiologic defense against overheating. Sweat glands, which are controlled by cholinergic sympathetic nerve fibers, secrete large quantities of hypotonic saline in response to heat stress. As the sweat reaches the skin, a cooling effect occurs as the fluid evaporates, and the blood that has been shunted from the interior to the surface of the skin is then cooled. The effectiveness of evaporative heat loss is determined by relative humidity. In high humidity, sweating represents a useless water loss and can lead to a dangerous state of dehydration and overheating [12].

In contradistinction, the initial result of cold exposure is a generalized reduction in skin temperature, which leads to cutaneous veno- and vasoconstriction [13]. A cold-induced increase in peripheral arterial resistance is initiated by beta-adrenergic receptor activation, which acts directly on blood vessel diameter. In addition, sudden cold exposure causes the release of norepinephrine, epinephrine, and cortisol from the adrenal gland [13]. The resultant reduction in peripheral blood flow redirects blood to the central circulation, which results in a rise in mean arterial pressure, cardiac output, and stroke volume.

Heat production via shivering thermogenesis is initiated once there is a significant reduction in body temperature. The contractile force generated by the shivering muscles may be 15% to 20% of that elicited during maximal voluntary muscle activation [13]. It is mediated by somatic nerves and requires an intact spinal cord and posterior hypothalamus [2]. Nonshivering thermogenesis, an increased metabolic heat production from sources other than muscular contraction, also occurs during cold stress. The sources in animals include both an elevated rate of aerobic metabolism of brown adipose tissue as well as the stimulating effects of metabolic hormones [14].

Alterations in autonomic nervous system function after spinal cord injury

Spinal cord injury results in a reduction or lack of autonomic control that is directly related to the level of injury. Spinal cord injury interrupts the connections between the supraspinal regulatory centers and the effector organs and interferes with both afferent and efferent signal transmission. Many of the major cardiovascular functions are associated with segmental outflow from several levels, such as the outflow to the heart or the splanchnic outflow. Sympathetic control of blood vessels in the limbs and skin, as well as sweat glands, tends to be regionalized to more limited levels of the spinal cord (see Table 2 for synopsis).

Supraspinal control of the SNS originates in the rostroventrolateral (RVL) medulla, which is the main sympathetic regulatory center in the CNS [15]. Descending sympathetic input from this supraspinal center travels through the cervical spinal cord and synapse via spinal interneurons with the

Table 2
Spinal cord anatomy of sympathetic and parasympathetic outflow

CNS or Spinal cord level	ANS division	Ganglion	Nerve	Organs innervated
Dorsal motor nucleus of cranial nerve X	PNS	Not applicable	Vagus nerve Cardiac nerves	Heart, lungs, abdominal viscera, ascending and transverse colon
T1–T4	SNS	Middle cervical and stellate	Cardiac nerves	Heart, Lungs
T3–L3 (but mainly T5-T9)	SNS	Superior mesenteric (but does not synapse)	Lesser splanchnic nerve	Adrenal medulla
T5–T11	SNS	Celiac and superior mesenteric	Greater and lesser splanchnic nerves	Abdominal viscera Ascending and transverse colon
L1–L3	SNS	Inferior mesenteric	Lumbar splanchnic nerves	Descending colon and rectum, kidney, bladder, uterus, external genitalia
S2–4	PNS	Not applicable	Pelvic splanchnic nerves	Descending colon and rectum, bladder, uterus, external genitalia

sympathetic preganglionic neurons starting at T1. Thus, spinal cord injury above T1 interrupts the conduction of signals from the medulla to the thoracic spinal cord. These changes are more significant with more severe injuries [16]. Autopsies findings in patients with cervical SCI and severe cardiovascular abnormalities showed marked loss of axons in the dorsal aspects of the lateral funiculus, which is thought to be the location of the descending vasomotor pathways [16,17].

The sympathetic innervation to the heart, including the myocardium, SA, and AV nodes, is from T1 to T4. Thus, injuries between T1 and T4 have partial innervation to the heart, and injuries below T4 gain complete innervation to the heart. Thus, if the level of injury is below T4, normal cardiac responses are maintained, but vascular tone and control of blood pressure will still be under local regulation. Because the parasympathetic innervation to the heart is via the vagus nerve, which does not travel in the spinal cord, the only supraspinal control of cardiac responses is parasympathetic in nature.

Sympathetic outflow to the splanchnic organs mainly originates from T5 to T9 via the greater splanchnic nerve to the celiac ganglion (although there are splanchnic efferents from T5 to L2). This outflow regulates most of the blood flow in the splanchnic circulation. Injuries below T5 have some ability to regulate splanchnic flow, with more control with distal levels of injury. Damage to the spinal cord above this outflow hinders the ability of the splanchnic beds to vasodilate, which allows blood to pool in the splanchnic circulation. This lack of compensatory response to an elevation in blood pressure is part of the pathogenesis of autonomic dysreflexia, which occurs in persons with SCI above T6.

The sympathetic efferents to the adrenal medulla are from T3 to L3, but the major outflow is T5 to T9. This innervation allows control of the release of epinephrine from the adrenal medulla, which is part of the normal response to exercise or stress. Thus, injuries above T9 will have an impaired adrenal response to exercise. Sympathetic efferents to the blood vessels of the lower extremities travel through the upper lumber sympathetic ganglia; thus, vasomotor responses of the lower extremity vessels are abnormal with levels of injury above T12. Only injuries below L1 have minimal effects of SNS dysregulation.

Sympathetic control of blood vessels in the limbs, skin, and sweat glands are more regionalized than the major outflows and functions listed above. Sweat glands receive dual innervation from both cholinergic and adrenergic fibers; however, cholinergic stimulation provokes the largest response [2,18]. Spinal segments T2 to T4 supply sweat glands on the head and neck, T2 to T8 to glands of the upper limbs, T6 to T10 to the trunk, and T11 to L2 to the lower extremities [2,18]. Autonomic dermatomes overlap several segments above and below the somatic levels.

After injuries above T1, with loss of supraspinal connections to the sympathetic nervous system, homeostasis is achieved via local and spinal reflex control. There is evidence that after SCI, spinal circuits are capable of generating some sympathetic activity [19]. Sympathetic preganglionic neurons show spontaneous activity after SCI in the absence of input and function as "spinal sympathetic interneurons" [20]. There is also peripheral alpha-adrenoceptor hyperresponsiveness, which is thought to contribute to the propensity for autonomic dysreflexia. Sympathovagal balance appears to be maintained, secondary to a decrease in parasympathetic activity that parallels the decline in sympathetic activity [21].

Sympathetic preganglionic neurons show morphologic changes after spinal cord injury because of denervation from a lack of descending input. This leads to low resting blood pressure, orthostatic hypotension, and loss of diurnal fluctuation of blood pressure [22]. This decrease in the diurnal variation of blood pressure in persons with cervical SCI is because normal nocturnal decreases in blood pressure do not occur [23]. In addition, the 24-hour plasma noradrenaline level in individuals with SCI also shows little diurnal variation. Interestingly, both sympathetic and parasympathetic preganglionic neurons in the lumbar and sacral spinal cord are less severely affected than those in the thoracic cord and seem to be more dependent on innervation from spinal interneurons for synaptic input [24].

Cardiovascular alterations immediately after spinal cord injury

In the first few minutes after SCI, there is a disruption in central sympathetic control caused by interruption of the descending pathways that travel in the spinal cord. Animal studies have found that within seconds to minutes after injury, there is a systemic pressor response that results from a burst of sympathetic activity and outflow of adrenaline from the adrenal glands [25]. In the feline model of SCI, compression of the cervical spinal cord causes a brief increase in both systolic and diastolic blood pressure, with corresponding bradycardia [26]. In addition, electrocardiogram changes include ventricular ectopy and a left ventricular strain pattern. Tibbs and colleagues [27] used a canine model in a series of studies showing that spinal cord transection creates an initial increase of norepinephrine, with associated hypertension, increased systemic vascular resistance, increased left ventricular ejection fraction, and bradycardia with escape arrhythmias [27–30]. Guha and Tator [31] used rats with a clip compression injury model, and showed that T1 SCI is characterized by a brief hypertensive peak (2 to 3 minutes in their model). All investigators noted that profound hypotension followed this initial hypertensive episode.

After this initial brief pressor response, studies of acute SCI in both humans and animals show an extended period of neurogenic shock characterized by hypotension, bradycardia, and hypothermia [32]. Neurogenic shock is a direct result of the loss of supraspinal control and reduction in sympathetic activity below the level of injury, which is substantiated by low plasma adrenaline, noradrenaline, and urinary metabolites after SCI [33]. Neurogenic shock is part of the spinal shock syndrome, which is the period after injury characterized by a marked reduction or abolition of sensory, motor, or reflex function of the spinal cord below the level of injury [34].

Studies in the feline model of SCI show markedly decreased cardiac sympathetic tone. The loss of direct sympathetic influence on the heart appears to be the primary reason for decreased cardiac output, with a marked decrease in both heart rate and contractility [35]. Hypotension and bradycardia also occurs in the rat model of SCI [36]. This is thought to be because of the strong cholinergic input from unopposed vagal tone leading to nitric oxide release and vasodilation [37]. In addition, vagal stimulation may also depress cardiac function by slowing atrioventricular conduction and altering the synchronicity of the atrial and ventricular contractions, which impairs ventricular filling. Also cholinergic influences depress atrial contractility by antagonizing adrenergic influences on the heart.

The extent and severity of the blood pressure and heart rate changes appears to correlate with the location and severity of the spinal cord injury. Lehmann and colleagues [38] studied 71 persons after SCI, and found that 68% of individuals with complete tetraplegia (21 of 31) had hypotension (defined as systolic blood pressure <90 mm Hg), whereas none of the motor incomplete tetraplegics nor paraplegics met the criteria for hypotension. Delineating the effects of acute sympathetic nervous system withdrawal from hemodynamic shock can be difficult, especially in patients with multitrauma. Thus management must take into consideration both scenarios.

The pathophysiology of acute SCI is thought to be in part caused by spinal cord ischemia. This ischemia may be caused by local factors such as the direct effects of the SCI and focal vasospasm, both of which lead to loss of autoregulation of spinal cord blood flow. In addition, systemic factors such as hypotension also lead to decreased spinal cord blood flow and perfusion. This is compounded by the effects of bradycardia, arrhythmias, reduced mean arterial pressure (MAP), reduced pulmonary vascular resistance (PVR), and decreased cardiac output. Several studies have looked at maintenance of adequate systolic blood pressure as an important way to improve prognosis after acute SCI, based on the reduction of cord ischemia [39].

Hypotension

In recently injured persons with cervical spinal cord injury, the supine MAP averages 57 mm Hg compared with 82 mm Hg in supine non–cord-injured persons [40].

In the recently published guidelines on blood pressure management after acute SCI, the conclusion based on review of existing Class III evidence is that providing blood pressure support to keep the MAP >85 to 90 mm Hg improves neurologic outcomes [39]. The duration of blood pressure support is not clear, and 5 to 7 days was chosen arbitrarily based on similar data in patients after traumatic brain injury. All articles describe the use of central venous pressure or Swan Ganz catheter monitoring to determine fluid status followed by initial volume resuscitation with crystalloid and then colloid (whole blood or plasma) as indicated. If MAP remains below 85 mm Hg, most studies describe the use of pressors, typically a beta-agonist, followed by an alpha-agonist. Another recent review looked at the intensive care unit management of SCI, and recommended close attention to invasive hemodynamic monitoring and volume replacement or use of pressors as indicated [41].

Tator and colleagues [42] studied 144 patients with SCI who were treated with close attention to the management of respiratory failure and aggressive treatment of hypotension with crystalloid and whole blood or plasma transfusion. They compared outcomes with a cohort of 358 patients who were treated at their center before institution of the above treatment principles. Overall morbidity and mortality were reduced, as were costs and length of stay; these improvements were attributed to the improved respiratory management and avoidance of hypotension.

Levi and colleagues [43] treated 50 patients who had acute cervical SCI with a protocol that focused on improved cardiac output and keeping MAP >90 mm Hg by use of invasive monitoring along with volume and pressor support. Thirty-one patients were Frankel A, eight patients were Frankel B, and 11 patients were Frankel C and D. Eighty two percent of patients had volume-resistant hypotension requiring pressor within the first 7 days of treatment, which was 5.5 times more common in those with motor complete injuries. These patients had a reduced peripheral vascular resistance index, with 58% having values below normal. Half the patients also had a reduced systemic vascular resistance index. The investigators noted that no patient with a motor complete injury and marked deficits in these vascular indices experienced neurologic recovery at 6 weeks.

Vale and colleagues [44] managed a cohort of 77 patients with acute SCI with invasive monitoring and blood pressure support to maintain a MAP >85 mm Hg for 7 days after injury. The average pretreatment MAP for the American Spinal Injury Association (ASIA) A cervical patient was 66 mm Hg. Nine of ten cervical ASIA A patients required pressor to meet the MAP goal, and 52% of the incomplete cervical injuries needed pressors. Only nine of 29 thoracic level patients needed pressors to meet the MAP goal of >85. Minimal morbidity was associated with the use of invasive monitoring or pressors. Reported outcomes were very good, with three of ten cervical ASIA A patients regaining ambulatory function, and 23 of 25 patients with incomplete cervical SCI were ambulatory at 1 year. The investigators reported improved neurologic outcomes based on this strategy, but without a control group it is difficult to tell.

Ball [45] discusses treatment of acute hypotension, which is caused by loss of vasomotor tone and pooling of blood in the peripheral and splanchnic vasculature. They recommend volume resuscitation of 1 to 2 L, with caution not to infuse excess volume in a normovolemic patient. Because of the interruption of the sympathetic cardioaccelerator fibers, the heart cannot compensate for the increased venous return with an increase in heart rate, thus, the only change that can occur is an increase in stroke volume (which may not be attainable). Thus, use of a vasopressor with both alpha- and beta-adrenergic actions (such as dopamine or norepinephrine) is ideal, to give the heart the chronotropic support as well as counteracting the lack of sympathetic tone to the vessels. This prevents complications associated with volume overload, including pulmonary edema.

Zach and colleagues [46] managed 117 patients with acute SCI, using central venous pressure monitoring and volume expansion to maintain blood pressure for 7 days. They reported that 62% of the patients with cervical injuries improved, with two patients improving by two grades and one patient by three grades. No patient with a cervical injury worsened, and 38% were unchanged. Patients who were admitted within 12 hours of injury were more likely to improve than those admitted later (after 48 hours). The study was limited by lack of a control or comparison group. The investigators concluded that early management and close attention to maintaining an acceptable blood pressure improved prognosis.

Wolf and colleagues [47] combined aggressive medical and surgical management of patients with acute cervical bilateral facet dislocations. Treatment included monitoring and maintenance of MAP above 85 mm Hg for 5 days in combination with immediate closed or open reduction of the cervical spine. They report improvement in 21% of patients with complete and 62% of patients with incomplete cervical injuries. The investigators concluded that their management protocol improved outcomes after acute cervical SCI. The study was limited by lack of a control group.

Bradycardia

Bradycardia often is seen in patients with cervical spinal cord injury because of a preponderance of vagal tone and a lack of descending sympathetic input. This bradycardia lasts for 2 to 6 weeks after injury; however, episodes of persistent bradycardia after that time may occur in severe injuries [48]. Lehmann and colleagues [38] studied 71 consecutive patients after SCI. All 31 with severe cervical SCI (Frankel A and B) had persistent bradycardia (<60 beats per minute). The severe cervical group also had more marked bradycardia (pulse <45); hypotension with systolic blood pressure of <90 mm Hg; supraventricular arrhythmias, predominantly atrial fibrillation; and primary cardiac arrest (16% versus 0 versus 0%). Twenty-nine percent of the severe cervical group required repeated injections of atropine or a transvenous pacer, whereas none in the other groups did.

In Lehmann and colleagues' [38] study, primary cardiac arrest occurred in five of 31 patients, and all were Frankel A. All had shown some cardiovascular abnormality, including hypotension and persistent bradycardia in all five, a need for pressor therapy in four, a need for atropine in three, and prior tachyarrhythmias and new AV block in two. Three of the cardiac arrests had a fatal outcome. The frequency of bradyarrhythmias peaked on day 4 after injury and subsided over the first 10 days. All observed abnormalities (including hypotension and bradycardia) resolved within 2 to 6 weeks. All these events are thought to be secondary to lack of sympathetic innervation to the heart in patients with cervical SCI. Evidence to support this includes the frequency of bradyarrhythmias in cervical SCI, low baseline serum catecholamines, a subnormal increase in heart rate with atropine, the prevention of bradyarrhythmias with low-dose sympathomimetics, and the ability of unopposed vagal tone to cause bradycardia, sinus arrest, AV block, and atrial fibrillation.

Severe bradycardia and sinus arrest have been reported to occur after vagal stimulation such as tracheal suctioning in tetraplegics [49–51]. Hypoxia stimulates a sympathetic response through the pulmonary inflation reflex and a vagal response through carotid body chemoreceptor activation [50]. Although in non–cord-injured individuals the sympathetic response dominates and produces tachycardia in the presence of hypoxia, in persons with cervical spinal cord injuries, the response to hypoxia is paradoxical bradycardia. This is thought to be caused by the lack of sympathetic tone that would normally counteract the rise in vagal tone with suctioning or other maneuvers (including defecation or even turning). The treatment of bradyarrhythmias with atropine is only partially and transiently effective, which is consistent with the lack of sympathetic tone as the cause rather than excessive parasympathetic tone. Use of low-dose isoproterenol was suggested by Lehmann and colleagues [38], which reportedly eliminated the sinus pauses.

The guidelines for implantation of permanent pacemakers in individuals with cervical spinal cord injuries and persistent cardiovascular abnormalities are not clear, and the literature in this area is limited to case reports. Ruiz-Arango and colleagues [52] reported three cases of patients with cervical SCI who required permanent pacemaker implantation. All cases were patients with injuries at C5 or above who had recurrent desaturation and prolonged mechanical ventilation, episodes of hypoxia leading to profound bradycardia and asystole, and cardiac arrhythmias requiring temporary pacing. In this case series, the most common arrhythmia was bradycardia, but patients also had AV block (first-degree and Mobitz II), atrial fibrillation, sinus arrest with sinus pauses, and asystole. In two of these patients, vagal stimulation triggered asystole necessitating resuscitation. Bilello reported on 83 patients with tetraplegia and divided them into the high cervical group (C1 to C5) and the low cervical group (C6 to C7) [25]. All patients had hypotension (systolic blood pressure <90) and bradycardia (heart rate <50), but 24% of the high group needed cardiovascular interventions including pressors, chronotropes, and cardiac pacing. Only 5% of the low group required cardiovascular interventions. Two patients in the high cervical group required permanent pacemakers.

Respiratory impairments

In addition to the cardiovascular consequences of spinal cord injury, which include hypotension and bradycardia, there are also pulmonary consequences of the loss of supraspinal sympathetic control. These cause respiratory impairments in addition to those created by the lack of innervation to respiratory musculature. The pulmonary vascular bed also has sympathetic innervation, and the lack of sympathetically mediated bronchodilation may exacerbate respiratory difficulties. In addition, neurogenic pulmonary edema occurs not uncommonly after acute SCI.

Neurogenic pulmonary edema is attributed to an immediate increase in blood pressure after SCI, with resultant increase in systemic and pulmonary vascular pressures. This increase results in a shift of blood from the high-resistance systemic circulation to the low-resistance pulmonary circulation [53]. In addition, aggressive fluid resuscitation is not uncommon because of the inability to gauge fluid status in an acutely injured patient with severe hypotension; thus, the patient may be hypervolemic [54]. Marked increases in pulmonary vascular pressures and in pulmonary blood volume then produce pulmonary edema because of the hydrostatic effect of increased pulmonary capillary pressure [55]. In addition, pulmonary hypertension and hypervolemia injure pulmonary blood vessels, altering pulmonary capillary permeability. After the transient systemic and pulmonary vascular hypertension subsides, the patient is left with abnormal pulmonary capillary permeability, so that pulmonary edema persists [53]. Neurogenic pulmonary edema has been reported to occur with autonomic dysreflexia, which supports the theory that a massive sympathetic discharge is the initiating event in neurogenic pulmonary edema [56].

The altered response of the pulmonary vascular bed after cervical SCI was studied by Levi and colleagues [43]. These investigators treated 50 patients with acute cervical SCI and noted that patients with a low pulmonary vascular resistance index (PVRI) were less likely to recover any neurologic function than patients with a higher pulmonary or systemic vascular resistance index. They also noted that these patients have a reduced response to conventional volume challenge within the pulmonary vasculature, which is improved with small amounts of dopamine. They hypothesized that the poor prognosis for patients with low PVRI is reflective of the severity of the SCI and that the pulmonary vascular bed is more sensitive to the sympathectomized effects of cervical SCI.

Schilero and colleagues found that subjects with tetraplegia had significantly reduced airway conductance, which increased significantly after inhaled ipratropium bromide [56a]. They hypothesized that the reduced baseline airway caliber was due to heightened vagomotor airway tone, due to interruption of sympathetic innervation to the lungs. The anticholinergic properties of the ipratropium act to decrease vagal tone to the airways and allow bronchodilation.

Postacute cardiovascular responses

Neuronal activity in the spinal cord neurons slowly returns after SCI, marking the emergence from spinal shock [57]. Spinal shock typically persists for 4 to 6 weeks, but there is still a lack of clarity regarding the definition of the end of spinal shock, because different reflexes tend to recover at different times. For example, the bulbocavernosus reflex returns within 24 to 48 hours after SCI, whereas deep tendon reflexes take 2 weeks to return after injury [19]. Several studies have noted the return of heart rate and blood pressure to near normal values within 5 to 7 days of lower cervical and upper thoracic SCI [58,59]. However, after the acute phase of SCI, alterations in cardiovascular function continue to exist because of the lack of central regulation of the autonomic nervous system.

In general, basal systolic and diastolic blood pressure in tetraplegics is about 15 mm Hg lower than that in normal subjects [50]. This is because of the interruption of supraspinal sympathetic input and is reflected by low levels of plasma noradrenaline and adrenaline. As would be expected, an inverse relationship between level of injury and blood pressure has been found, which is thought to be the result of the lack of sympathetic vasoconstrictor influences below the level of injury [60]. In persons with chronic tetraplegia, supine blood pressure is lower than in non–cord-injured persons with loss of the nocturnal circadian fall of blood pressure [61]. Krum and colleagues [62] studied 10 persons with cervical spinal cord injuries compared with 10 immobilized controls, measuring blood pressure and heart rate variability over a 24-hour period. Nighttime blood pressures were the same in both groups, but daytime blood pressures were higher in non–cord-injured persons. These variations were not associated with postural changes. The findings suggest that the normal diurnal variation in sympathetic activity is absent in persons with tetraplegia.

Other cardiovascular alterations after SCI include changes in heart and cardiac output. Individuals with mid-thoracic cord injuries have elevated heart rates at rest and with activity. In addition, they have lower stroke volumes at rest and with activity than non–cord-injured people [63]. This elevated heart rate may be a compensatory mechanism for the reduced stroke volume, which is caused by decreased venous return from regions below the level of injury. This reduction in venous return is caused by both lack of effective muscle pumping action and lack of sympathetic vasoconstrictor tone [8].

In persons with chronic SCI, vascular adaptations are seen, including 30% reduction in femoral artery diameter, with a reduction in blood flow and doubling of stress levels in the femoral artery. These adaptations occur within the first 6 weeks after injury, with extensive reductions in femoral diameter and leg volume and increased basal shear rate levels and flow-mediated dilation [64]. The change in limb volume caused by muscle atrophy parallels the time course of the arterial changes and is proportional, suggesting a functional link between muscular and arterial adaptations.

de Groot and colleagues [65] found that the dimensions of the left ventricle, left atrium, and vena cava are all reduced in persons with cervical SCI. However, systolic and diastolic functions are not altered, suggesting that the changes in the cardiac structure are adaptive. These changes are hypothesized to be caused by a variety of factors including vascular atrophy and reduced total blood volume, reduced cardiac filling, stroke volume and cardiac output, and decreased preload caused by pooling of blood in the lower extremities, low systolic blood pressure, and lower heart rate. These may result in lower left ventricular (LV) wall stress and subsequent cardiac atrophy. Nash found that LV myocardial atrophy is common in persons with chronic tetraplegia but that exercise could cause remodeling and an increase in LV mass [66].

Changes in circulating catecholamines

Free plasma catecholamine measurements are used to assess current sympathetic nervous system activity because of their short half-life. Plasma noradrenaline levels reflect sympathetic nerve functioning, whereas plasma adrenaline levels reflect adrenomedullary function [32,67,68]. Individuals with chronic tetraplegia have low basal levels of plasma noradrenaline and adrenaline [69,70]. Those individuals with injuries between T1 and T5 also have low levels of adrenaline, indicating impaired release of catecholamines from the adrenal medulla [69,71]. Individuals with injuries below T5 actually have levels of plasma catecholamines that are higher than non–cord-injured persons [72]. With exercise, persons with cervical-level injuries do not have augmentation of catecholamines, those with lesions from T1 to T5 have increased noradrenaline but not adrenaline, and those with lesions below T5 have an increase in both catecholamines [72]. This fact is again consistent with the known spinal level of innervation of the sympathetic outflow to the adrenal medulla.

Orthostatic hypotension

Blood pressure control depends on tonic activation of the sympathetic nervous system via descending input from supraspinal structures [19]. In non–cord-injured persons, assumption of upright posture is associated with pooling of blood in the lower extremities, which reduces cardiac output. This causes a decline in blood pressure, which is sensed by the aortic and carotid sinus baroreceptors. This causes a decrease in the rate of inhibitory afferent action potentials to the medullary vasomotor center via the glossopharyngeal and vagus nerves [2]. In response, there is sympathetic activation via descending spinal tracts, which causes vasoconstriction and also results in parasympathetic inhibition [32].

SCI interrupts the descending sympathetic input from the rostroventrolateral medulla, which is excitatory in nature. Without this tonic input, there is low resting blood pressure, loss of blood pressure autoregulation, and disturbed reflex control [73]. Reduced blood volume in the intrathoracic veins leads to decreased venous return, decreased ventricular end-diastolic filling pressure and stroke volume, and decreased cardiac output and arterial blood pressure [74–76]. In persons with SCI above T6, there is loss of vasoconstriction in the splanchnic bed, which contributes to loss of blood pressure autoregulation. Even in patients injured below T6, there is still loss of reflex vasoconstriction in the skeletal muscle bed, which may lead to a degree of orthostatic hypotension [60]. In addition, persons with paralysis of the lower extremity musculature loose the beneficial effects of the venous pumping action of active muscle contraction, thus contributing to venous pooling. All of these changes contribute to orthostatic hypotension after SCI.

Orthostatic hypotension is a decrease in systolic blood pressure of more than 20 mm Hg or a decrease in diastolic blood pressure of more than 10 mm Hg with upright posture or head-up tilt to 60° for at least 3 minutes [7]. This hypotension is typically accompanied by symptoms that are not necessarily related to absolute blood pressure. Symptoms of hypotension include fatigue or weakness, dizziness, light-headedness, blurred vision, dyspnea, and nausea [77,78]. In one study, 41% of cord-injured persons with orthostatic hypotension were asymptomatic, but 74% of spinal cord injured persons had orthostasis [79]. Orthostasis is severe acutely but persists for some patients chronically and may in fact worsen many years after injury [77].

Persons with spinal cord injury tolerate orthostasis well, perhaps because of changes in cerebral autoregulation that maintain cerebral blood flow and oxygenation despite greater decrease in MAP and stroke volume than noncord injured [80,81]. Typically, there is not a loss of consciousness with orthostasis, except in recently injured persons with tetraplegia or those with chronic tetraplegia after a period of recumbency. Studies in persons with tetraplegia have discovered the ability to autoregulate cerebral perfusion at lower systemic blood pressures. In the baboon model, cervical sympathectomy allows cerebral artery vasodilation and regulation of cerebral perfusion pressure at lower blood pressure levels than before sympathectomy.

There is a slight increase in heart rate during head-up tilt because of decreased baroreceptor activity causing a reduction in vagal tone. However, the heart rate does not typically go above 100 beats per minute because of lack of an intact sympathetic nervous system [82]. This effect is different from that in non–cord-injured individuals, who may become quite tachycardic with hypotensive episodes. Plasma noradrenaline levels do not increase with head-up tilt as expected because of the lack of ability to activate the sympathetic nervous system reflexively in response to a fall in blood pressure. However, there are a variety of other mechanisms that help the person with tetraplegia adapt to orthostatic challenges. The release of renin occurs independently of sympathetic stimulation, probably secondary to the decrease in renal perfusion pressure [82]. This results in the formation of angiotensin II, which is not only a vasoconstrictor but also facilitates peripheral NA release and the release of aldosterone from the adrenal cortex. Aldosterone serves to retain sodium and water, which increases intravascular volume [83]. Vasopressin (antidiuretic hormone) also is released, which causes fluid retention and decreased urine output during prolonged head-up tilt.

The return of lower extremity spasticity can counter the lower extremity venous pooling and reduces the incidence of orthostasis in those with chronic SCI. Other mechanisms that decrease the degree of orthostatic hypotension experienced by persons with chronic SCI include vigorous renal vasoconstriction and some autonomy of spinal vasomotor reflexes [19]. The management of orthostasis is discussed in detail in the review by Claydon and colleagues [84].

Temperature regulation

Although central temperature mechanisms are unaffected by spinal cord injury, there is impairment in the ability to regulate body temperature because of the loss of hypothalamic thermoregulatory control below the level of the injury. In addition, there is interruption of the afferent pathways from the peripheral temperature receptors below the level of SCI. In persons with spinal cord injury above T6, there is a complete loss of shivering, thermoregulatory sweating, and no peripheral circulatory adjustment below the lesion. Spinal cord–injured individuals have lower core temperatures in the cold than non-SCI individuals, resulting in the term *partial poikilotherms* [85]. There is some evidence of spinal reflex–mediated sweating, but this remains a matter of debate. Wallin and colleagues [86] found that changes in ambient temperature did not change the firing rate of sympathetic neurons, thus, leading to the conclusion that sympathetic thermoregulatory reflexes do not occur at the spinal level in humans. In paraplegics, deep or central temperature receptors sensitive to cold are able to initiate shivering above the level of the SCI. These receptors can act independently of the temperature of the skin above the SCI [87].

Summary

The autonomic nervous system plays a key role in the regulation of many physiologic processes mediated by supraspinal control from centers in the CNS. Spinal cord injury is associated with alterations in autonomic regulation, with level of injury playing a key role in the subsequent derangements that occur. Above T1, SCI causes a complete disruption of the sympathetic pathways and results in a variety of problems including bradycardia, neurogenic pulmonary edema, arrhythmias, and hypotension. SCI above T6 causes an altered splanchnic outflow, which causes hypotension and altered vascular regulation. Even persons with injuries below T6 have changes in cardiovascular response as consequences of the altered ANS regulation. In addition, persons with SCI have changes in circulating catecholamines, and many have persistent orthostasis as well as impaired temperature regulation, which are chronic issues. Thus, the role of autonomic dysfunction in persons with SCI is crucial to understand because many aspects of the altered physiology seen in these individuals are directly caused by ANS dysregulation.

References

[1] Mohrman D, Heller L. Chapter 9: Regulation of arterial pressure. In: Lange cardiovascular physiology. United States of America: McGraw-Hill Companies; 2006.
[2] Downey J, Myers SJ, Gonzalez EG, et al. The Physiological basis of rehabilitation medicine. 2nd edition. Boston: Butterworth-Heinemann; 1994.
[3] Appenzeller O, Oribe E. Autonomic anatomy, histology and neurotransmission. In: The autonomic nervous system: an introduction to basic and clinical concepts. 5th edition. New York: Elsevier; 1997. p. 2–8.
[4] Bonica JJ. Autonomic innervation of the viscera in relation to nerve block. Anesthesiology 1968;29(4):793–813.
[5] Loewy AD, Spyer KM. Central regulation of autonomic functions. New York: Oxford University Press; 1990.
[6] Janes RD, Brandys JC, Hopkins DA, et al. Anatomy of human extrinsic cardiac nerves and ganglia. Am J Cardiol 1986;57(4):299–309.
[7] Glenn MB, Bergman SB. Cardiovascular changes following spinal cord injury. Top Spinal Cord Inj Rehabil 1997;2(4):47–53.
[8] Collins HL, Rodenbaugh DW, DiCarlo SE. Spinal cord injury alters cardiac electrophysiology and increases the susceptibility to ventricular arrhythmias. Prog Brain Res 2006;152: 275–88.
[9] Mohrman D, Heller L. Chapter 7: Vascular control. In: Lange cardiovascular physiology: McGraw-Hill Companies; 2006.
[10] Simon E. Temperature regulation: The spinal cord as a site of extrahypothalamic thermoregulatory functions. Rev Physiol Biochem Parmacol 1974;71:1–76.
[11] Downey RJ, Downey JA, Newhouse E, et al. Hyperthermia in a quadriplegic: evidence for a peripheral action of haloperidol in malignant neuroleptic syndrome. Chest 1992;101: 1728–30.
[12] Macardle WD, Katch Frank I, Katch Victor L. Exercise physiology: energy, nutrition and human performance. 4th edition. Baltimore: Williams & Wilkins; 1996.
[13] Stocks JM, Taylor NA, Tipton MJ, et al. Human physiological responses to cold exposure. Aviat Space Environ Med 2004;75(5):444–57.
[14] Toner MM, McArdle WD. Human thermoregulatory responses to acute cold stress with special reference to water immersion. vol I. New York: Oxford University Press; 1996.
[15] Krassioukov AV, Fehlings MG. Effect of graded spinal cord compression on cardiovascular neurons in the rostro-ventro-lateral medulla. Neuroscience 1999;88(3):959–73.
[16] Krassioukov A. Which pathways must be spared in the injured human spinal cord to retain cardiovascular control? Prog Brain Res 2006;152:39–47.
[17] Furlan JC, Fehlings MG, Shannon P, et al. Descending vasomotor pathways in humans: correlation between axonal preservation and cardiovascular dysfunction after spinal cord injury. J Neurotrauma 2003;20(12):1351–63.

[18] Quinton P. Sweating and its disorders. Annu Rev Med 1983;34:429–52.
[19] Krassioukov A, Claydon VE. The clinical problems in cardiovascular control following spinal cord injury: an overview. Prog Brain Res 2006;152:223–9.
[20] Schramm LP. Spinal sympathetic interneurons: their identification and roles after spinal cord injury. Prog Brain Res 2006;152:27–37.
[21] Grimm DR, De Meersman RE, Almenoff PL, et al. Sympathovagal balance of the heart in subjects with spinal cord injury. Am J Physiol 1997;272(2 Pt 2):H835–42.
[22] Teasell RW, Arnold JM, Krassioukov A, et al. Cardiovascular consequences of loss of supraspinal control of the sympathetic nervous system after spinal cord injury. Arch Phys Med Rehabil 2000;81(4):506–16.
[23] Legramante JM, Raimondi G, Massaro M, et al. Positive and negative feedback mechanisms in the neural regulation of cardiovascular function in healthy and spinal cord-injured humans. Circulation 2001;103(9):1250–5.
[24] Llewellyn-Smith IJ, Weaver LC, Keast JR. Effects of spinal cord injury on synaptic inputs to sympathetic preganglionic neurons. Prog Brain Res 2006;152:11–26.
[25] Bilello JF, Davis JW, Cunningham MA, et al. Cervical spinal cord injury and the need for cardiovascular intervention. Arch Surg 2003;138(10):1127–9.
[26] Eidelberg EE. Cardiovascular response to experimental spinal cord compression. J Neurosurg 1973;38(3):326–31.
[27] Tibbs PA, Young B, McAllister RG, et al. Studies of experimental cervical spinal cord transection. Part I: hemodynamic changes after acute cervical spinal cord transection. J Neurosurg 1978;49(4):558–62.
[28] Tibbs PA, Young B, McAllister RG Jr, et al. Studies of experimental cervical spinal cord transection. Part III: effects of acute cervical spinal cord transection on cerebral blood flow. J Neurosurg 1979;50(5):633–8.
[29] Tibbs PA, Young B, Todd EP, et al. Studies of experimental cervical spinal cord transection. Part IV: effects of cervical spinal cord transection on myocardial blood flow in anesthetized dogs. J Neurosurg 1980;52(2):197–202.
[30] Tibbs PA, Young B, Ziegler MG, et al. Studies of experimental cervical spinal cord transection. Part II: plasma norepinephrine levels after acute cervical spinal cord transection. J Neurosurg 1979;50(5):629–32.
[31] Guha A, Tator CH. Acute cardiovascular effects of experimental spinal cord injury. J Trauma 1988;28(4):481–90.
[32] Bravo G, Guizar-Sahagun G, Ibarra A, et al. Cardiovascular alterations after spinal cord injury: an overview. Curr Med Chem Cardiovasc Hematol Agents 2004;2(2):133–48.
[33] Claus-Walker J, Halstead LS. Metabolic and endocrine changes in spinal cord injury: II (section 1). Consequences of partial decentralization of the autonomic nervous system. Arch Phys Med Rehabil 1982;63(11):569–75.
[34] Ditunno JF, Little JW, Tessler A, et al. Spinal shock revisited: a four-phase model [see comment]. Spinal Cord 2004;42(7):383–95.
[35] Yardley CP, Fitzsimons CL, Weaver LC. Cardiac and peripheral vascular contributions to hypotension in spinal cats. Am J Physiol 1989;257(5 Pt 2):H1347–53.
[36] Hall ED, Wolf DL. Post-traumatic spinal cord ischemia: relationship to injury severity and physiological parameters. Cent Nerv Syst Trauma 1987;4(1):15–25.
[37] Bravo G, Rojas-Martinez R, Larios F, et al. Mechanisms involved in the cardiovascular alterations immediately after spinal cord injury. Life Sci Feb 2001;68(13):1527–34.
[38] Lehmann KG, Lane JG, Piepmeier JM, et al. Cardiovascular abnormalities accompanying acute spinal cord injury in humans: incidence, time course and severity. J Am Coll Cardiol 1987;10(1):46–52.
[39] Blood pressure management after acute spinal cord injury. Neurosurgery 2002;50(3 Suppl): S58–62.
[40] Mathias CJ, Christensen NJ, Frankel HL, et al. Cardiovascular control in recently injured tetraplegics in spinal shock. Q J Med 1979;48(190):273–87.

[41] Management of acute spinal cord injuries in an intensive care unit or other monitored setting. Neurosurgery 2002;50(3 Suppl):S51–7.

[42] Tator CH, Rowed DW, Schwartz ML, et al. Management of acute spinal cord injuries. Can J Surg 1984;27(3):289–93.

[43] Levi L, Wolf A, Belzberg H. Hemodynamic parameters in patients with acute cervical cord trauma: description, intervention, and prediction of outcome. Neurosurgery 1993;33(6): 1007–16.

[44] Vale FL, Burns J, Jackson AB, et al. Combined medical and surgical treatment after acute spinal cord injury: results of a prospective pilot study to assess the merits of aggressive medical resuscitation and blood pressure management. J Neurosurg 1997;87(2): 239–46.

[45] Ball PA. Critical care of spinal cord injury. Spine 2001;26(24 Suppl):S27–30.

[46] Zach GA, Seiler W, Dollfus P. Treatment results of spinal cord injuries in the Swiss Paraplegic Centre of Basle. Paraplegia 1976;14(1):58–65.

[47] Wolf A, Levi L, Mirvis S, et al. Operative management of bilateral facet dislocation. J Neurosurg 1991;75(6):883–90.

[48] Gilgoff IS, Ward SL, Hohn AR. Cardiac pacemaker in high spinal cord injury. Arch Phys Med Rehabil 1991;72(8):601–3.

[49] Zipnick RI, Scalea TM, Trooskin SZ, et al. Hemodynamic responses to penetrating spinal cord injuries. J Trauma 1993;35(4):578–82.

[50] Mathias CJ. Bradycardia and cardiac arrest during tracheal suction–mechanisms in tetraplegic patients. Eur J Intensive Care Med 1976;2(4):147–56.

[51] Frankel HL, Mathias CJ, Spalding JM. Mechanisms of reflex cardiac arrest in tetraplegic patients. Lancet 1975;2(7946):1183–5.

[52] Ruiz-Arango AF, Robinson VJB, Sharma GK. Characteristics of patients with cervical spinal injury requiring permanent pacemaker implantation. Cardiol Rev 2006;14(4):e8–11.

[53] Theodore J, Robin ED. Speculations on neurogenic pulmonary edema (NPE). Am Rev Respir Dis 1976;113(4):405–11.

[54] Karlsson AK. Autonomic dysfunction in spinal cord injury: clinical presentation of symptoms and signs. Prog Brain Res 2006;152:1–8.

[55] Phanthumchinda K, Khaoroptham S, Kongratananan N, et al. Neurogenic pulmonary edema associated with spinal cord infarction from arteriovenous malformation. J Med Assoc Thai 1988;71(3):150–3.

[56] Kiker JD, Woodside JR, Jelinek GE. Neurogenic pulmonary edema associated with autonomic dysreflexia. J Urol 1982;128(5):1038–9.

[56a] Schilero GJ, Grimm DR, Bauman WA, et al. Assessment of airway caliber and bronchodilator responsiveness in subjects with spinal cord injury. Chest 2005;127(1):149–55.

[57] Gondim FAA, Lopes ACA Jr, Oliveira GR, et al. Cardiovascular control after spinal cord injury. Curr Vasc Pharmacol 2004;2(1):71–9.

[58] Krassioukov AV, Weaver LC. Reflex and morphological changes in spinal preganglionic neurons after cord injury in rats. Clin Exp Hypertens 1995;17(1–2):361–73.

[59] Maiorov DN, Weaver LC, Krassioukov AV. Relationship between sympathetic activity and arterial pressure in conscious spinal rats. Am J Physiol 1997;272(2 Pt 2):H625–31.

[60] Mathias CJ. Orthostatic hypotension: causes, mechanisms, and influencing factors. Neurology 1995;45(Suppl 5):S6–11.

[61] Nitsche B, Perschak H, Curt A, et al. Loss of circadian blood pressure variability in complete tetraplegia. J Hum Hypertens 1996;10(5):311–7.

[62] Krum H, Louis WJ, Brown DJ, et al. Diurnal blood pressure variation in quadriplegic chronic spinal cord injury patients. Clin Sci 1991;80(3):271–6.

[63] Jacobs PL, Mahoney ET, Robbins A, et al. Hypokinetic circulation in persons with paraplegia. Med Sci Sports Exerc 2002;34(9):1401–7.

[64] de Groot PC, Bleeker MW, van Kuppevelt DH, et al. Rapid and extensive arterial adaptations after spinal cord injury. Arch Phys Med Rehabil 2006;87(5):688–96.

[65] de Groot PC, van Dijk A, Dijk E, et al. Preserved cardiac function after chronic spinal cord injury. Arch Phys Med Rehabil 2006;87(9):1195–200.
[66] Nash MS, Bilsker S, Marcillo AE, et al. Reversal of adaptive left ventricular atrophy following electrically-stimulated exercise training in human tetraplegics. Paraplegia 1991;29(9): 590–9.
[67] Peronnet F, Beliveau L, Boudreau G, et al. Regional plasma catecholamine removal and release at rest and exercise in dogs. Am J Physiol 1988;254(4 Pt 2):R663–72.
[68] Jensen-Urstad M, Svedenhag J, Sahlin K. Effect of muscle mass on lactate formation during exercise in humans. Eur J Appl Physiol Occup Physiol 1994;69(3):189–95.
[69] Schmid A, Huonker M, Stahl F, et al. Free plasma catecholamines in spinal cord injured persons with different injury levels at rest and during exercise. J Auton Nerv Syst 1998; 68(1–2):96–100.
[70] Levin BE, Martin BF, Natelson BH. Basal sympatho-adrenal function in quadriplegic man. J Auton Nerv Syst 1980;2(4):327–36.
[71] Schmid A, Halle M, Stutzle C, et al. Lipoproteins and free plasma catecholamines in spinal cord injured men with different injury levels. Clin Physiol 2000;20(4):304–10.
[72] Schmid A, Huonker M, Barturen JM, et al. Catecholamines, heart rate, and oxygen uptake during exercise in persons with spinal cord injury. J Appl Physiol 1998;85(2):635–41.
[73] Mathias CJ, Frankel HL. Autonomic disturbance in spinal cord lesions. Oxford: Oxford Medical Publications; 1992.
[74] Faghri PD, Yount JP, Pesce WJ, et al. Circulatory hypokinesis and functional electric stimulation during standing in persons with spinal cord injury. Arch Phys Med Rehabil 2001; 82(11):1587–95.
[75] Ten Harkel AD, van Lieshout JJ, Wieling W. Effects of leg muscle pumping and tensing on orthostatic arterial pressure: a study in normal subjects and patients with autonomic failure. Clin Sci 1994;87(5):553–8.
[76] Jacobsen TN, Nielsen HV, Kassis E, et al. Subcutaneous and skeletal muscle vascular responses in human limbs to lower body negative pressure. Acta Physiol Scand 1992;144(3): 247–52.
[77] Frisbie JH, Steele DJ. Postural hypotension and abnormalities of salt and water metabolism in myelopathy patients. Spinal Cord 1997;35(5):303–7.
[78] Sclater A, Alagiakrishnan K. Orthostatic hypotension. A primary care primer for assessment and treatment. Geriatrics 2004;59(8):22–7.
[79] Illman A, Stiller K, Williams M. The prevalence of orthostatic hypotension during physiotherapy treatment in patients with an acute spinal cord injury. Spinal Cord 2000;38(12): 741–7.
[80] Houtman S, Colier WN, Oeseburg B, et al. Systemic circulation and cerebral oxygenation during head-up tilt in spinal cord injured individuals. Spinal Cord 2000;38(3):158–63.
[81] Gonzales F, Chang JY, Banovac K, et al. Autoregulation of cerebral blood flow in patients with orthostatic hypotension after spinal cord injury. Paraplegia 1991;29:1–7.
[82] Mathias CJ. Orthostatic hypotension and paroxysmal hypertension in humans with high spinal cord injury. Prog Brain Res 2006;152:231–43.
[83] Schmitt JK, Koch KS, Midha M. Profound hypotension in a tetraplegic patient following angiotensin-converting enzyme inhibitor lisinopril. Case report. Paraplegia 1994;32(12): 871–4.
[84] Claydon VE, Steeves JD, Krassioukov A. Orthostatic hypotension following spinal cord injury: understanding clinical pathophysiology. Spinal Cord 2006;44(6):341–51.
[85] Sawka MN, Latzka WA, Pandolf KB. Temperature regulation during upper body exercise: able-bodied and spinal cord injured. Med Sci Sports Exerc 1989;21(5 Suppl):S132–40.
[86] Wallin BG, Stjernberg L. Sympathetic activity in man after spinal cord injury. Outflow to skin below the lesion. Brain 1984;107(Pt 1):183–98.
[87] Downey JA, Chiodi HP, Darling RC. Central temperature regulation in the spinal man. J Appl Physiol 1967;22(1):91–4.

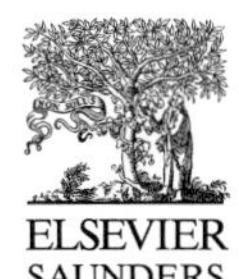
ELSEVIER
SAUNDERS

Phys Med Rehabil Clin N Am
18 (2007) 297–316

PHYSICAL MEDICINE
AND REHABILITATION
CLINICS OF
NORTH AMERICA

Preventive Care in Spinal Cord Injuries and Disorders: Examples of Research and Implementation

Frances M. Weaver, PhD[a,b,c,*],
Sherri L. LaVela, MPH, MBA[a,b,d,e,*]

[a]*Center for Management of Complex Chronic Care (CMC3), Health Services Research (151H), VA Hospital, Hines, IL 60141, USA*
[b]*SCI Quality Enhancement Research Initiative, Department of Veterans Affairs (DVA), Health Services Research (151H), VA Hospital, Hines, IL 60141, USA*
[c]*Neurology Department, Northwestern University, Feinberg School of Medicine, 303 E. Chicago Avenue, Chicago, IL 60611, USA*
[d]*US National Institutes of Health, National Institute on Aging, 1747 West Roosevelt Road, Chicago, IL 60608, USA*
[e]*Center for Research on Health and Aging, Institute for Health Research and Policy, 1747 West Roosevelt Road, Chicago, IL 60608, USA*

Prevention is a primary goal of medical care. For individuals with chronic impairments, such as those with spinal cord injuries and disorders (SCD [unless otherwise specified, the abbreviation SCD will refer to individuals with spinal cord injuries and/or disorders]), prevention is an even more important goal, because illness often is complicated by the existing disability. Health care providers and individuals with SCD need to be very concerned with prevention of common problems, such as, for example, influenza, because the literature indicates that persons with spinal cord injuries who contract influenza have a much higher risk of dying from complications than those in the general population [1]. Issues such as smoking and obesity, which are affected by individual lifestyle and behaviors, take on greater complexity in persons with SCD who have respiratory impairments and greater challenges with physical activity and diet. Research indicates that

This work was supported by the Spinal Cord Injury Quality Enhancement Research Initiative, Research Coordinating Center, Hines VA Hospital.

* Corresponding authors. Department of Veterans Affairs, Hines VA Hospital, HSR&D P.O. Box 5000 (151H), Midwest Center for Health Services & Policy Research, 5th Avenue and Roosevelt Road, Hines, IL 60141-5000.

E-mail addresses: frances.weaver@va.gov (F.M. Weaver); sherri.lavela@va.gov (S.L. LaVela).

doi:10.1016/j.pmr.2007.03.002

individuals with disabilities are less likely to receive preventive care services and screenings than the general population [2,3]. This chapter provides information on current prevalence proportions of several preventable conditions for individuals with SCD, presents the current evidence regarding prevention of these illnesses and conditions, and then provides examples of how use to implementation strategies to increase the use of evidence-based preventive care in individuals with SCD.

Prevalence of common conditions

The major causes of death in the United States are chronic diseases, including heart disease and cancer [4]. These and many other serious health problems are thought to disproportionately affect individuals with SCD and to affect them at earlier ages than the general population. A recent survey of veterans with SCD was conducted to assess the prevalence of conditions or diseases, characterize the nature and extent of health behaviors, assess the provision and use of preventive health services, and to determine factors and characteristics that influenced health promotion behaviors in individuals with SCD [5]. This survey replicated items from the Behavioral Risk Factor Surveillance System (BRFSS) survey, which was developed to provide data for health planning and policy and to serve as an infrastructure for behavioral surveillance [6]. The BRFSS is an ongoing annual surveillance system supported by the Centers for Disease Control and Prevention (CDC) that is used to collect data on the behaviors and conditions that place adults at risk for chronic illnesses, injuries, and preventable infectious diseases that are the primary causes of morbidity and mortality in the United States. A limitation to these public data is that information specific to individuals with several types of disabilities is not available. The survey (SCD_BRFSS), using items from the BRFSS survey [7], was fielded to individuals with SCD to obtain disability-specific information.

The 2003 cross-sectional, prospective SCD_BRFSS survey was distributed to members of the Paralyzed Veterans of America (PVA) (including those who receive health care at Veterans Health Administration [VHA] facilities and elsewhere). Survey questions were derived from the CDC BRFSS questionnaire (core and optional modules, BRFSS) [7]. Respondents were men (97%), white (82%), and had completed some college or technical school (72%), and 58% were married. On average, they were 60 years of age, nearly a quarter lived alone (24%), and only 10% were employed for wages. More than half had a paraplegic-level injury (52%), had been injured for an average of 24 years, and had an average age at injury of 36 years.

The prevalence of several conditions is presented below, followed by use of preventive health services with references to the recommended guidelines for each service as documented by appropriate organizations such as the US Preventive Services Task Force; National Heart, Lung, and Blood Institute; American Cancer Society; and the Advisory Committee on Immunization

Practices (ACIP). Each preventive measure was examined in terms of appropriate timing and age of receipt according to the guidelines.

Prevalence proportions from the SCD_BRFSS survey were compared with the national 2003 population-based CDC BRFSS survey data [8]. Data were examined overall and by age categories for several conditions and diseases for which prevention can have a significant impact. Findings are presented in Table 1.

Cholesterol and blood pressure

Notably more respondents with SCD than those in the general population reported having high blood pressure (note that autonomic dysreflexia may complicate this method of self-report) (49% versus 26%, respectively) and high cholesterol (47% versus 30%, respectively). Not surprisingly, prevalence increased with age in both groups; however, as age increased, differences between groups declined. Studies using clinical data have found that although about 10% of the US population has high-density lipoprotein (HDL) values <35 mg/dL, 24% to 40% of individuals with tetraplegia have been found to have depressed HDL values [9,10]. Among persons with all levels of SCD, approximately 25% have elevated low-density lipoprotein (LDL) levels [11]. In another study, Weaver and colleagues [12] concluded that providers need guidelines to address prevention and treatment of these prevalent conditions in SCD and point out that these also serve as risk factors for several other chronic conditions such as cardiovascular disease and diabetes.

Table 1
Comparison of selected disease/condition prevalence in veterans with SCD versus general population BRFSS data

	Veterans with SCD	General population data[a]
Diabetes[b]	—	—
Overall	19.39	6.7
Aged 55–64	20.75	12.7
Aged 65+	25.08	15.5
High blood pressure[c]	—	—
Overall	48.90	25.6
Aged 55–64	50.68	41.9
Aged 65+	61.70	53.0
High cholesterol[c]	—	—
Overall	47.03	30.2
Aged 55–64	50.43	43.9
Aged 65+	49.40	43.9

[a] Median percent from nationwide BRFSS data.
[b] BRFSS 2002 nationwide data.
[c] BRFSS 2001 nationwide data; 2002 not available.

Diabetes

Self-reported diabetes was more prevalent in patients with SCD than in the general population overall (19% versus 7%) and for those aged 55 to 64 (21% versus 13%) and aged 65 and older (25% versus 16%) according to the SCD_BRFSS and the CDC 2003 BRFSS. Other studies have reported rates of diabetes from 13% to 22% in individuals with SCD [13,14]. LaVela and colleagues [15] found that one fourth of persons with SCD and diabetes reported that diabetes affected their eyes or that they had retinopathy (25%), and 41% had foot sores that took more than 4 weeks to heal. These rates are higher than reported rates for the population in general. Unique challenges related to common risk factors for diabetes in the SCD population (eg, inactivity, decreased muscle mass), and the consequences of diabetes and slower healing suggest that guidelines on diabetes prevention and care management specific to SCD would be advantageous. In the interim, a reasonable strategy would be to follow the existing guidelines for diabetes screening and management for the general population in SCD (eg, VHA/Department of Defense clinical Practice Guideline for Management of Diabetes Mellitus in Primary Care; http://www.oqp.med.va./gov/cpg/cpg.htm accessed 1/23/2007).

In addition to the areas covered in the SCD_BRFSS survey, the literature discusses other areas in which careful attention to and development of preventive measures to improve and maintain the health of persons with SCD would be highly beneficial. These include the growing epidemic of obesity, infections, and some cancers.

Obesity

Obesity is a significant problem for individuals with disabilities. Although 15% of the general population is considered obese, 25% of persons with disabilities have been identified as being obese [16]. In addition, individuals with mobility difficulties had the greatest risk of being obese. George and colleagues [17] reported that sedentary men with spinal cord injuries had an average body fat percentage of 25% compared with 17% for weight-matched, able-bodied men when measured by hydrodensitometry. Spungen and colleagues [18] found that persons with SCD were 13% ± 1% fatter per unit of body mass index (BMI) (based on fat to lean body mass) than an able-bodied group, suggesting that ideal body weight charts should be adjusted when evaluating individuals with SCD. In a sample of veterans with SCD, Weaver and colleagues [12] found that 20% had a BMI greater than or equal to 30 kg/m^2, putting them into the obese category but cautioned that this is likely an underestimation of obesity in SCD. The ability to address obesity prevention in persons with SCD is hampered by not only intrinsic complexities such as difficulty exercising in high-level tetraplegia, but also by a lack of guidelines for health care providers on how to help persons with SCD lose weight and exercise.

Infection

Individuals with SCD have a high lifelong risk for systemic infection [19]. Infection is the most common reason for rehospitalization and emergency room visits [20,21] and a primary cause of death for persons with SCD [22]. Common infections in SCD include pneumonias, urinary tract infections, and infections from pressure ulcers. LaVela and colleagues [23] found that urinary tract infections and bloodstream infections were the most common nosocomial infections in veterans with SCD. Further, the overall number of nosocomial infections in this population (36.1 per 1000 patient days) was higher than what has been reported in the literature in various populations (ranges from 2.2 to 15 per 1000 patient days) [24–26]. Persons with SCD are more likely to be hospitalized than those in the general public, and the risk of contracting a nosocomial infection increases with longer lengths of hospital stays, thus increasing the risk of infection in SCD.

Prevention is of utmost importance in this population because persons with SCD often spend more time in a hospital setting (at risk for hospital-acquired infections) [20], are more likely to rely on medical equipment and devices [27,28], and may have more skin infections while hospitalized because of multiple changes in skin morphology [29] and susceptibility to pressure ulcers [30] than those in other populations. Specific guidelines to prevent or reduce infection occurrence in SCD are beginning to emerge. For example, the CDC has identified SCD as a high-risk condition for influenza vaccination [31], prioritizing receipt of this preventive measure among this population. Respondents to the SCD_BRFSS survey were slightly less likely to be vaccinated against influenza and more likely to be vaccinated against pneumonia than those in the general population (67% versus 70%; and 73% versus 64%; respectively).

Cancer (select examples)

Bladder cancer

Individuals with SCD are at increased risk of bladder cancer; this cancer is more likely to be diagnosed at a later stage and is less likely to be amenable to surgical treatment and more likely to result in death [32]. Surveillance is more difficult because it is common to have other symptoms or signs that may be indicative of cancer in the general population but not in persons with SCD. For example, hematuria is rare in the general population but may occur quite frequently in people who use catheters. Several retrospective studies have found that the rate of squamous cell bladder cancer is higher in individuals with SCD who have used long-term indwelling catheters for 8 or more years to manage their bladders [33–35]. Individuals with SCD are 15.2 times more likely to have bladder cancer than those in the general population [33]. However, this cancer is rare, so the numbers in those with SCD, although higher than in the general population, are low.

The Consortium for Spinal Cord Medicine recently published a clinical practice guideline on bladder management for persons with spinal cord injuries [36]. Although the guideline recommends the use of intermittent catheterization for bladder management, when possible, to limit complications, there are a number of reasons why this strategy is not possible in some individuals, including those who are unable to catheterize themselves, those who have poor cognition or lack motivation, those who have high fluid intake, and those with bladder anatomy abnormalities. In these individuals, it is important to address other risk factors, such as smoking, and to monitor them for the possible occurrence of cancer.

Prostate cancer

Uncertainty exists and the literature is inconclusive regarding risk for prostate cancer in patients with SCD. Some studies have found that testosterone levels that are usually low in individuals with SCD may be protective against prostate cancer [37,38]. Other studies have reported that prostatic inflammation puts persons with SCD at increased risk for prostate cancer [39,40]. Although some research has reported that the incidence of prostate cancer [41] and the proportion of individuals with prostate cancer is lower in persons with SCD than the general population, it is more likely to be diagnosed at a more advanced stage and grade [42]. As the lifespan for persons with SCD approaches that of the general population, prostate cancer is likely to become a more clinically significant disease in these men [43]. Additional research is necessary to understand the usefulness of supplementary screening programs for this population.

Colorectal cancer

It is unclear whether the risk for colorectal cancer is higher in persons with SCD. One study found a two to six times higher incidence of colorectal cancer in SCD than in the able-bodied population [44]. Another study reported that the incidence is the same as in the normal population but noted that the diagnosis often was delayed in SCD [45]. Problems such as constipation and sensory deficits [46] may put persons with SCD at greater risk for colorectal cancer. In addition, surveillance is challenging in SCD, because blood in the stool (one of the main screening tests) is common in people who do digital stimulation with their bowel program, making the specificity and sensitivity of such tests very different in the SCD population. Also, many of the lifestyle and behaviorally based risk factors for colorectal cancer (eg, physical inactivity, obesity) [47] are more prevalent in persons with SCD. General recommendations for colon cancer screening exist, and at least one study has made specific recommendations for individuals with SCD (described below) [48].

Issues of preventive care in SCD

Advances in treatment and technology have improved such that people with SCD have increasingly longer life expectancies [49,50]. As aging occurs in this cohort, they are at increased risk for secondary conditions and other diseases, making health prevention and maintenance necessary elements of their lifelong care [51].

An important component of prevention is the use of screening tests and health promotion campaigns. However, health promotion strategies and wellness programs traditionally have not been a major part of the rehabilitation process in individuals with SCD [52–54]. Disability-related concerns may displace preventive health during routine health care visits [54,55]. More recently it has been recognized that, just as in the general population, the overall lifetime health profile of an individual with SCD is the result of interaction between health care (and disability) management and lifestyle practices and behaviors [56]. Therefore, it is believed that secondary conditions and premature mortality in the SCD population may be influenced by positive changes in lifestyle behaviors [57] and attentiveness to prevention.

The 2003 SCD_BRFSS survey [5] provided information on the use of preventive services among individuals with SCD. Some of these are discussed in detail below; findings are presented in Table 2.

Healthy People 2010 objectives include increasing the proportion of adults who have had their blood cholesterol checked within the preceding 5 years, with a target of 80% [57]. The National Cholesterol Education Program of the National Heart, Lung, and Blood Institute recommends that all persons aged >20 years have their cholesterol checked at least once every 5 years. SCD_BRFSS survey findings indicated that 92% of adults with SCD have had their cholesterol checked at least once in the prior 5 years.

The ACIP recommends annual influenza vaccination for persons at high risk for medical complications from influenza, including individuals with SCD, regardless of age [31]. The ACIP also recommends the pneumococcal polysaccharide vaccine (PPV) for persons 65 and older and persons at increased risk for pneumococcal disease or its complications [58]. This includes previously unvaccinated persons and persons who have not received the vaccine within 5 years (and were less than 65 years of age at the time of vaccination). The Healthy People 2010 target for noninstitutionalized adults aged 65 years and older for annual influenza and a single PPV is 90%, and for noninstitutionalized high-risk adults aged 18 to 64 years the target is 60% [57]. Individuals with SCD exceeded these targets; the SCD_BRFSS findings indicate that 67% of individuals with SCD had received an annual influenza vaccination, and 73% had ever received a pneumonia vaccine.

The US Preventive Services Task Force strongly recommends that clinicians screen men and women 50 years of age or older for colorectal cancer. A 10-year interval has been recommended for colonoscopy. Shorter intervals (5 years) have been recommended for flexible sigmoidoscopy because of lower sensitivity, but there is no direct evidence with which to determine the optimal interval [59]. Stiens and colleagues [48] recommend that a sigmoidoscopy or colonoscopy be performed every 3 to 5 years in persons

Table 2
Use of preventive health care services

Preventive health test/measure	SCD_BRFSS results (%)
Cholesterol checked within the past 5 years for patients ≥20 years of age[a] (n = 3630)	92.29
Influenza vaccination within the past year[b] (n = 4221)	67.24
Pneumonia vaccine—ever received[c] (n = 3855)	73.28
Colon screening in persons >50 years[d] (n = 3335)	—
Within past 5 years	58.68
Within past 10 years	66.15
Prostate tests (PSA and/or DRE) in men 50–70 (45–70 in African American)[e]	—
PSA past year (n = 2246)	52.09
DRE past year (n = 2305)	54.92
PSA *or* DRE past year (n = 2278)	69.10
PSA *and* DRE past year (n = 2240)	38.48
Mammogram within past year for women ≥40[f] (n = 112)	65.18
Pap Smear within past year for women 18–70[g] (n = 110)	87.27
Within past 3 years (n = 110)	61.82

Abbreviations: DRE, digital rectal examination; PSA, prostate-specific antigen.

[a] The National Cholesterol Education Program of the National Heart, Lung, and Blood Institute recommends that all persons aged ≥20 years have their cholesterol checked at least once every 5 years.

[b] ACIP recommends annual influenza vaccination in persons 50 and older and persons at high risk for medical complications from influenza.

[c] ACIP recommends pneumococcal polysaccharide vaccine for persons 65 and older and persons at increased risk for pneumococcal disease or its complications. This includes previously unvaccinated persons and persons who have not received vaccine within 5 years (and were less than 65 years of age at the time of vaccination). All persons who have unknown vaccination status should receive one dose of vaccine.

[d] The U.S. Preventive Services Task Force (USPSTF) strongly recommends that clinicians screen men and women 50 years of age or older for colorectal cancer. A 10-year interval has been recommended for colonoscopy. Shorter intervals (5 years) have been recommended for flexible sigmoidoscopy because of lower sensitivity, but there is no direct evidence with which to determine the optimal interval. Case-control studies have suggested that sigmoidoscopy every 10 years may be as effective as sigmoidoscopy performed at shorter intervals.

[e] The USPSTF found good evidence that prostate-specific antigen (PSA) screening can detect early-stage prostate cancer but mixed and inconclusive evidence that early detection improves health outcomes. If early detection improves health outcomes, the population most likely to benefit from screening will be men aged 50 to 70 who are at average risk and men older than 45 who are at increased risk (African American men and men with a family history of a first-degree relative with prostate cancer). Older men and men with other significant medical problems who have a life expectancy of fewer than 10 years are unlikely to benefit from screening. The American Cancer Society believes that health care professionals should offer the PSA blood test and DRE yearly.

[f] The USPSTF recommends screening mammography, with or without clinical breast examination, every 1 to 2 years for women aged 40 and older. The American Cancer Society recommends that women aged 40 and older should have a screening mammogram every year.

[g] The USPSTF found good evidence that screening with Pap smears reduces incidence of and mortality from cervical cancer. Direct evidence to determine the optimal starting and stopping age and interval for screening is limited. Indirect evidence suggests most of the benefit can be obtained by beginning screening within 3 years of onset of sexual activity or age 21 (whichever comes first) and screening at least every 3 years. The USPSTF found limited evidence to determine the benefits of continued screening in women older than 65. The yield of screening is low in previously screened women older than 65 because of the declining incidence of high-grade cervical lesions after middle age. New American Cancer Society recommendations suggest stopping cervical cancer screening at age 70.

with SCD who are 50 years of age and older. Using SCD_BRFSS data, the receipt of colon screening (either sigmoidoscopy or colonoscopy) within the previous 5 and 10 years in respondents with SCD aged 50 and older was examined. The Healthy People 2010 target for adults aged 50 years and older who have ever received a sigmoidoscopy is 50% [57]. The findings of the SCD_BRFSS indicate that 59% of individuals with SCD underwent a colon screening (sigmoidoscopy or colonoscopy) in the last 5 years and 66% within the prior 10 years.

Significant evidence exists in many of the health care areas identified above as to how to best manage individuals to prevent or reduce the likelihood of secondary complications.

Use of evidence-based care guidelines leads to improved patient outcomes [60,61]. One way that these evidence-based findings have been disseminated is through the publication of clinical practice guidelines.

Clinical practice guidelines

A clinical practice guideline (CPG) provides a set of evidence-based recommendations on how to manage or treat a particular condition or problem. These guidelines are usually published by highly reputable medical societies or academic groups and involve a thorough review of the literature on the topic of concern. Furthermore, the evidence is graded based on how it was obtained. There are several methods for grading the strength of evidence. One of the more commonly used methods was developed by Sackett [62]. Research papers and studies are graded on a 1 to 5 scale: 1 = large randomized trials with clear-cut findings and low risk of error; 2 = small randomized trials with less certain results and greater risk; 3 = nonrandomized studies or contemporaneous controls; 4 = nonrandomized trials using historical controls; and 5 = case series with no controls. In some cases, a recommendation will be made that is not based on strong evidence but is supported by the consensus of experts on the CPG panel.

In the area of spinal cord injury (SCI), 21 organizations have formed a consortium to develop CPGs. These organizations include the Paralyzed Veterans of America, the American Association of Neurological Surgeons, the American Physical Therapy Association, and the Department of Veterans Affairs (among others). Using a steering committee to identify topics for CPGs and nominate panel members for development of the CPG, the Consortium for Spinal Cord Medicine (CSCM) has published nine CPGs. Consumer input is also sought for each of the guidelines. Topics include bowel care, bladder care, autonomic dysreflexia, depression, respiratory management, outcomes after traumatic SCI, upper limb preservation, prevention of thromboembolism, and pressure ulcers (these are available at www.pva.org). Five guidelines also have consumer guides. Many of the recommendations are focused on the prevention of further disability or complications. Unfortunately, the evidence is weak in many areas of SCD, so recommendations are either drawn from other populations for which evidence exists or are based on expert consensus and strength of the panel's opinion (ie, low, moderate or strong agreement with recommendation). Even in cases in which the evidence is not strong, the CPG provides a set of recommendations that allow for the standardization of care and documentation so that patient outcomes can be monitored and compared.

Implementation of evidence-based care: examples in prevention

Despite widespread dissemination of CPGs and strong evidence for following certain prevention care practices, patients often do not receive evidence-based care. There are many possible reasons including lack of knowledge on the part of providers or patients, resistance to change, limitations or barriers within the health care system (eg, a particular drug is not on the hospital formulary), lack of decision support, limits in the computer infrastructure (eg, a computer reminder does not exist), or lack of support from administration to make changes [63,64]. Below are three examples of efforts to increase the use of evidence-based care for prevention in veterans with SCD: respiratory vaccinations, smoking cessation, and neurogenic bowel care. This type of work is called *implementation research*. "Implementation research is the scientific study of methods to promote the systematic uptake of clinical research findings and other evidence-based practices into routine practice, and hence to improve the quality and effectiveness of health care. It includes the study of influences on healthcare professional and organizational behaviour." (from http://www.implementationscience.com/info/about/ accessed 12/12/2006).

Respiratory vaccinations

Individuals with SCD are at high risk for respiratory complications because their respiratory muscles often are weak, which impairs their ability to cough. This in turn leads to less effective clearing of pulmonary secretions, and, as a result, morbidity and mortality from respiratory-related illnesses are higher than in the general population [49,65]. The 2005 annual report from the Model Spinal Cord Injury System (MSCIS) indicates that almost 22% of deaths in SCI were caused by diseases of the respiratory system, of which, 71.7% were pneumonias [66]. Further, DeVivo and colleagues [1] reported that persons with SCD who contract influenza or pneumonia are 37 times more likely to die from influenza or pneumonia complications than comparable persons from the general population. Using the National Death Index files, respiratory-related illnesses were found to account for 12% of deaths in veterans with SCD (4% were specifically caused by pneumonia) [67]. This difference in rates may in part be because of the somewhat different populations examined; the MSCIS cohort includes all traumatic SCI cases and includes a large percentage of cases in which cause of death is missing, whereas the VHA cohort is comprised of persons with both traumatic and nontraumatic spinal impairments and is an older cohort than MSCIS, and, for the cohort examined, cause of death was available for almost all veterans over a 2-year period. Nonetheless, respiratory-related illnesses and death continue to be a significant concern in SCD.

It is well accepted that influenza vaccination is a successful method to decrease the risk of respiratory illness. Vaccination is effective in reducing the likelihood of contracting influenza and pneumonia, lessening the severity of respiratory illnesses and decreasing the likelihood of death from complications of influenza or pneumonia [68–70]. The effectiveness of the influenza vaccination has been seen in various age groups and populations [70–71] including persons with SCD [72]. The CSCM's CPG on "Respiratory management following SCI" [73] does recommend influenza vaccination, but there is no discussion of how best to implement this in SCD. Until recently, SCD was not identified as a high-risk group for vaccination. The VHA began including SCD as one of its high-risk categories for vaccination in their annual influenza policy memos regarding vaccination in 2002, and the CDC added neuromuscular diseases including SCI in their high-risk category in 2005 [31]. Specifically, the recommendation states "that persons with any condition (eg, cognitive dysfunction, spinal cord injuries, seizure disorders, or other neuromuscular disorders) that can compromise respiratory function or the handling of respiratory secretions or that can increase the risk for aspiration be vaccinated against influenza."

A medical record review of documented influenza vaccinations in a sample of veterans with SCD followed up in VHA SCI Centers in the mid-1990s found rates of vaccination to be low ($\leq$25%) in those 65 years of age and older [74]. In contrast, vaccination rates in the general veteran population age 65 and older were significantly higher (71%). Subsequently, VHA developed a performance management system in which a set of performance indicators were used to monitor how well VHA facilities were providing preventive and chronic care services. Influenza vaccination was included as one of the prevention indicators for both the general veteran population and for veterans with SCD. In fiscal year 2001, the vaccination indicator became a performance measure, and VHA facilities were held accountable for their performance. However, there continued to be a significant gap in vaccination rates between the general veteran population and veterans with SCD.

The SCI Quality Enhancement Research Initiative (QUERI), one of 10 centers in VHA focused on implementation research, began to examine why vaccine rates continued to be lower in the SCD population. A mailed survey was administered to veterans with SCD at eight VHA SCI centers. Barriers to vaccination were identified from the perspective of the veteran including a poor understanding of the seriousness of influenza and its complications and of the vulnerability that an individual with SCD has to respiratory complications [75]. During this pilot work, letters were mailed to a sample of veterans with SCD reminding them to get vaccinated and providing information about their increased risk for respiratory complications because of their spinal impairment. Results indicated that self-reported vaccination rates were significantly higher for veterans who received mailed reminders than for those who did not receive reminders (60.5% versus 54.3%; $P<.01$; [76]).

This pilot work was used to develop a 2-year national implementation study involving all 23 VHA SCI centers. The intervention was a multistrategy effort based on a review of the literature on effective vaccination strategies and the earlier pilot work. It was targeted to veterans, providers, and the health care system and included veteran and provider reminder letters and education, use of computerized clinical reminders, and nurse standing orders [77]. Monthly calls were held with participating centers to discuss the status of vaccination activities. During these calls it became evident that (1) computerized clinical reminders only targeted veterans with SCD if they were age 65 or older and (2) a nurse standing order was a local facility policy decision. Working with VHA's clinical applications coordinators who develop and manage computerized reminders, the vaccine reminder diagnosis taxonomy was modified so that it would include all veterans with an SCD diagnosis, regardless of age. The taxonomy was in place before the second year of the study.

The baseline influenza vaccination rate was 33% in fiscal year (FY) 2001. The percentage of veterans with SCD who reported receiving vaccinations increased to 62.5% in year 1 (FY02) and 67.4% in the second year ($P = .004$); for those <50 years old, rates increased from 50% to 54% between the first and second years. These numbers are quite impressive when you consider that among persons with diabetes (a long-standing high-risk group for vaccination), approximately 56% of those between the ages of 50 and 64 years and only 37.8% of those aged 18 to 49 years were vaccinated in 2002 [68]. Although it was not possible to directly assess the impact of increased rates of influenza vaccination on patient outcomes, estimates of impact based on studies of non-SCI populations can be determined. Vaccination rates in veterans with SCD have increased from 25% to 72% in 10 years. This increase is likely to have resulted in 41 fewer deaths per year caused by respiratory complications of influenza, 25% fewer days of missed work or reduced functioning, and reductions in annual outpatient visits and hospital admissions by 44% and 37%, respectively [78].

Smoking cessation

Between one half and two thirds of persons with acute SCD have respiratory complications [79,80]. These include atelectasis, pneumonia, and respiratory failure. These continue to be frequent complications during chronic SCD as well. The negative effect of smoking on pulmonary function among individuals with SCD is evident. In a survey of 180 individuals with SCD, individuals with tetraplegic-level injuries who were current smokers reported having greater phlegm and phlegm plus cough than nonsmokers

[81]. Linn and colleagues [82] found that smokers who had a tetraplegic-level injury were more at risk for decline in pulmonary function than smokers with paraplegia and that this risk increased with age. However, as is true in the general population, quitting smoking also reduces the long-term risk for obstructive lung diseases in SCD. Another study found that respiratory morbidity was related to tetraplegic injury, number of cigarettes smoked per day, and the interaction between cigarettes smoked and excessive alcohol use [83]. Although these studies point to greater risk in tetraplegia, the harms caused by smoking are relevant for those with paraplegic-level impairments as well.

Studies have consistently linked tobacco use with a number of chronic diseases, including pulmonary and cardiovascular conditions. A review of deaths in veterans with SCD using the National Death Index files found that almost 12% died of respiratory-related illnesses or conditions, including 4% for pneumonia or influenza, whereas heart diseases accounted for 25% of all deaths, and malignant neoplasms accounted for 22% of deaths [67]. The National MSCIS data indicate that heart disease is the leading cause of mortality (35% to 46%) for persons surviving >30 years after SCI and among those over age 60 [22,50] and accounted for 12% of deaths overall [66]. In fact, cardiovascular disease mortality rates in the SCD population are more than twice that in the nondisabled population [84].

Smoking is another example for which there is very strong evidence that quitting improves health, yet rates remain unacceptably high for the veteran SCD population. The CPG on "Respiratory management following SCI" [73] does mention the need to educate patients about smoking cessation, but no specific recommendation is made. Studies of veterans with SCD have found that approximately one third are current smokers (EPRP FY02-05) despite the high incidence of respiratory impairments in this population. In comparison, the prevalence of smoking in the general US adult population is approximately 21% [85]. The rate at which VHA health care providers counsel or advise a person to quit smoking has improved significantly from 58% (FY03) to 96% (FY06) for veterans with SCD, yet the percentage of smokers has not declined in the last several years.

As with the respiratory vaccine work described above, SCI QUERI investigators identified potential barriers to smoking cessation with input from providers and veterans with SCD. The leveling off of the rate of decrease in smoking in veterans with SCD may be attributable, at least in part, to patient barriers. In a recent survey of veterans with SCD it was found that current smokers are younger and more likely to have alcohol problems, depression, or posttraumatic stress than nonsmokers with SCD [86]. Reasons for smoking included relaxation (10%), tension reduction (9%), and psychological addiction (9%). Only a small number of participants reported having tried available smoking cessation interventions, and most rated these as not being very helpful. On the other hand, more than half of those surveyed could be classified as having a low degree of nicotine dependence. Findings suggest, therefore, that the veterans surveyed were relatively light smokers who would be expected to quit more successfully than heavier smokers.

Other potential barriers exist at the provider and system levels. A recent study of national trends in tobacco cessation treatment in VHA reports low use of smoking cessation aids [87]. Only 7% of smokers in VHA received a prescription for nicotine replacement therapy (NRT). Two thirds of those who received a prescription received the nicotine patch, 25% received bupropion, and fewer than 10% were prescribed nicotine gum. VHA changed its policy regarding prescription of NRT in August 2003 (VHA Directive 2003-042). The original policy required that NRT only be prescribed if an individual was willing to attend a smoking cessation program. The 2003-042 directive indicated that smoking cessation medication should be made available to all smokers interested in quitting, regardless of whether they are willing to attend a cessation program or clinic. However, as recently as June 2006, some VHA SCI centers and clinics were operating under the old policy and were not being allowed to prescribe NRT to their patients. The VHA's Office of Quality and Performance added a new tobacco performance measure for FY07 to assess whether providers offer medications/NRT as part of their smoking cessation treatment [88].

Lack of access to care is both a patient- and a system-level barrier. At one VHA SCI center, a group of psychologists learned that only one veteran with SCD had enrolled in the primary care smoking cessation clinic. The major barrier identified by the psychologists was physical access to the clinic (eg, location, transportation, mobility limits). As a result, the psychologists created a smoking cessation clinic on the SCI unit. During the first year 17 veterans with SCD enrolled; in the second year 12 more enrolled. Long-term quit rates (6%) were similar to those in the general population [89]. This experience suggests that involving psychologists more systematically on the SCI unit or clinic is feasible, acceptable to patients, and effective.

Other efforts are being made to address smoking cessation in SCD at the patient, provider, and system levels including greater use of behavioral interventions and greater focus on the lenient attitudes of staff toward patient smoking (zero tolerance goal).

Neurogenic bowel management

The third implementation example describes increasing the use of the neurogenic bowel CPG [90]. After an SCD, neurogenic bowel dysfunction is common. Problems include fecal incontinence, difficulties with evacuation, and other complications that affect patient quality of life and can lead to life-threatening situations [91]. Up to three quarters of individuals with an SCD will experience fecal incontinence [92]. Use of an effective bowel management program can minimize these problems and complications.

The CSCM published a clinical practice guideline entitled "Neurogenic bowel management in adults with spinal cord injury" in 1998 [90] with the goal of improving evidence-based care for management of neurogenic bowel that would minimize complications and negative outcomes. Researchers conducted a study to examine provider adherence to the neurogenic bowel CPGs during two time periods: after distribution of the guidelines and after targeted implementation of six of the 31 recommendations [93]. Using an expert panel of clinicians, other providers, and research methodologists, six of the recommendations with the greater potential for impact were translated into specific performance measures that could be assessed using existing data (eg, medical records, administrative data). These recommendations included documentation of bowel care programs (#17), assessment of function (#4), content of patient history (#2), content of physical examination under medical review criteria (#3), (patient) education and competence in bowel management (#30 + 31), and colorectal cancer screening (#21). As has been documented elsewhere with other guidelines, dissemination of the neurogenic bowel guidelines had very little impact on adherence rates to the guidelines over the preguideline period.

The investigators developed a series of strategies to facilitate implementation of the guidelines by providers [93]. First, they conducted focus groups at each of the six study sites to learn about facilitators and barriers to implementing the guidelines. This feedback led to the use of two strategies: (1) development and dissemination of a standardized documentation template for bowel care (for inpatients) and (2) development of a patient-mediated intervention that emphasized the importance of patients in managing their neurogenic bowel. These strategies were associated with significant increases in adherence for three of the six guidelines. Recommendations 2 and 3 (documentation of patient history and physical examination) were followed some of the time before implementation, and documentation for both increased after implementation. Documentation of bowel care programs (#17) was poor before implementation, but increased significantly, most likely because of the provision of a standardized documentation tool. Although adherence was 40% after implementation, there continues to be considerable room for improvement. Adherence to recommendations 4, 30, and 31 was high at baseline, so there was less room for improvement, and these rates did not change. Although the investigators also tried to assess neurogenic bowel outcomes as a function of adherence to guidelines, many of the outcomes of interest were not always reliably collected. Some problems, such as hemorrhoids or rectal bleeding, were so common in this population that they were not charted routinely. The presumption is that effective use of guidelines results in improved patient outcomes. Unfortunately, given the limits in the data, this could not be ascertained in this study.

Summary

Prevention is an important component of the care of persons with SCD. These individuals are at increased risk for some common illnesses and have added risks for spinal cord–related problems. The use of evidence-based findings through tools like CPGs and evidence-based recommendations is key to improving patient outcomes and preventing avoidable illnesses and complications. Barriers exist to provision of preventive care, thus, providers and individuals with SCD must identify and overcome these barriers to ensure that high-quality care is delivered in a timely manner. Implementation research offers methods to increase use of evidence-based care.

Acknowledgments

The authors thank Dr. Bridget Smith and Ms. Charlesnika Evans for their early reviews of this manuscript.

References

[1] DeVivo MJ, Black KJ, Stover SL. Causes of death during the first 12 years after spinal cord injury. Arch Phys Med Rehabil 1993;74:248–54.
[2] Chan L, Houck PM, Rosenblatt RA, et al. Influenza vaccinations of Washington State Medicare beneficiaries seen by physiatrists in the outpatient setting in 1994. Arch Phys Med Rehabil 1998;79:599–603.
[3] Iezzoni LI, McCarthy EP, Davis RB, et al. Use of screening and preventive services among women with disabilities. Am J Med Qual 2001;16(4):135–44.
[4] Hoyert DL, Heron MP, Murphy SL, et al. Deaths: final data for 2003. Natl Vital Stat Rep 2006;54(13):1–120.
[5] LaVela SL. The epidemiology of health behavior and health status in individuals with SCI&D and multiple sclerosis. Project funded by: Department of Veterans Affairs, Health Services Research and Development, 2003–2004.
[6] Behavioral Risk Factor Surveillance System Survey User's Guide. Atlanta (GA): US Department of Health and Human Services, Centers for Disease Control and Prevention; 1998.
[7] Behavioral Risk Factor Surveillance System Survey (questionnaire). Atlanta (GA): US Department of Health and Human Services, Centers for Disease Control and Prevention; 2002/2003.
[8] Behavioral Risk Factor Surveillance System Survey (data). Atlanta (GA): U.S. Department of Health and Human Services, Centers for Disease Control and Prevention; 2003.
[9] Bauman WA, Adkins RH, Spungen AM, et al. The effect of neurological deficit on oral glucose tolerance in persons with chronic spinal cord injury. Spinal Cord 1999;37(11): 765–71.
[10] Brenes G, Dearwater S, Shapera R, et al. High density lipoprotein cholesterol concentrations in physically active and sedentary spinal cord injured patients. Arch Phys Med Rehabil 1986; 67:445–50.
[11] Bauman WA, Spungen AM, Zhong YG, et al. Depressed serum high density lipoprotein cholesterol levels in veterans with spinal cord injury. Paraplegia 1992;30:697–703.
[12] Weaver FM, Collins E, Kurichi J, et al. Prevalence of obesity and high blood pressure in veterans with spinal cord injuries and disorders: a retrospective review. Am J Phys Med Rehabil 2007;86(1):22–9.
[13] Bauman WA, Adkins RH, Spungen AM, et al. Is immobilization associated with abnormal lipoprotein profile? Observations from a diverse cohort. Spinal Cord 1999;37:485–93.
[14] Bauman WA, Spungen AM. Disorders of carbohydrate and lipid metabolism in veterans with paraplegia or quadriplegia: a model of premature aging. Metabolism 1994;43:749–56.

[15] LaVela SL, Weaver FM, Goldstein B, et al. Diabetes Mellitus in individuals with a spinal cord injury or disorder. J Spinal Cord Med 2006;29(4):387–95.
[16] Weil E, Wachterman M, McCarthy EP, et al. Obesity among adults with disabling conditions. JAMA 2002;288(10):1265–8.
[17] George CM, Wells CL, Dugan WL. Validity of hydrodensitometry for determination of body composition in spinal injured subjects. Hum Biol 1988;60:771–80.
[18] Spungen AM, Atkins RH, Steward CA, et al. Factors influencing body composition in persons with spinal cord injury: a cross-sectional study. J Appl Physiol 2003;95:398–407.
[19] Waites KB, Canupp KC, Chen Y, et al. Bacteremia after spinal cord injury in initial versus subsequent hospitalizations. J Spinal Cord Med 2001;24(2):96–100.
[20] Meyers AR, Branch LG, Cupples A, et al. Predictors of medical care utilization by independently living adults with spinal cord injuries. Arch Phys Med Rehabil 1989;70: 471–6.
[21] Davidoff G, Schultz S, Lieb T, et al. Rehospitalization after initial rehabilitation for acute spinal cord injury: incidence and risk factors. Arch Phys Med Rehabil 1990;71:121–4.
[22] Devivo M, Stover S. Long term survival and causes of death. In: Stover SL, DeLisa JA, Whiteneck GG, editors. Spinal cord injury clinical outcomes from the model systems. Gaithersburg (MD): Aspen Publishers; 1995. p. 289–313.
[23] LaVela SL, Evans CT, Miskevics S, et al. Long-term outcomes form nosocomial infections in persons with spinal cord injuries and disorders. Am J Infect Control, in press.
[24] Josephson A, Karanfil L, Alonso H, et al. Risk-specific nosocomial infection rates. Am J Med 1991;91(Suppl 3b):131S–7S.
[25] Richards MJ, Edwards JR, Culver DH, et al. Nosocomial infections in combined medical-surgical intensive care units in the United States. Infect Control Hosp Epidemiol 2000;21: 510–5.
[26] Urrea M, Pons M, Serra M, et al. Prospective incidence study of nosocomial infections in a pediatric intensive care unit. Pediatr Infect Dis J 2000;22:490–3.
[27] Gilmore DS, Schnick DG, Young MN, et al. Effect of external urinary collection system on colonization and urinary tract infections with Pseudomonas and Klebsiella in men with spinal cord injury. J Am Paraplegia Soc 1992;15:155–7.
[28] Mansel JK, Norman JR. Respiratory complications and management of spinal cord injuries. Chest 1990;97(6):1446–52.
[29] Frost FS, Pien LC, et al. The immune system and inflammatory response in persons with SCI. In: Lin VW, Cardenas DD, Cutter NC, editors. Spinal cord medicine: principles and practice. New York: Demos Medical Publishing; 2003. p. 213–20.
[30] Salzberg CA, Byrne DW, Cayten CG, et al. Predicting and preventing pressure ulcers in adults with paralysis. Adv Wound Care 1998;115:237–46.
[31] CDC-ACIP. Prevention and control of influenza: recommendations of the Advisory Committee on Immunization Practices (ACIP). MMWR Recomm Rep 2005;54(RR08):1–40.
[32] Vaidyanathan S, Mansour P, Soni BM, et al. The method of bladder drainage in spinal cord injury patients may influence the histological changes in the musoca of neuropathic bladder—a hypothesis. BMC Urol 2002;2:1–7.
[33] Groah SL, Weitzenkamp DA, Lammertse DP, et al. Excess risk of bladder cancer in spinal cord injury: evidence for an association between indwelling catheter use and bladder cancer. Arch Phys Med Rehabil 2002;83(3):346–51.
[34] Stonehill WH, Dmochowski RR, Patterson AL, et al. Risk factors for bladder tumors in spinal cord injury patients. J Urol 1996;155:1248–50.
[35] West DA, Cummings JM, Longo WE, et al. Role of chronic catheterization in the development of bladder cancer in patients with spinal cord injury. Urology 1999;53: 292–7.
[36] Consortium for Spinal Cord Medicine (CSCM). Bladder management for adults with spinal cord injury: A clinical practice guideline for health-care providers. Washington, DC: Paralyzed Veterans of America; 2006.

[37] Benaim EA, Montoya JD, Saboorian MH, et al. Characterization of prostate size, PSA and endocrine profiles in patients with spinal cord injuries. Prostate Cancer Prostatic Dis 1998;1: 250–5.

[38] Huang TS, Wang YH, Lee SH, et al. Impaired hypothalamuspituitary-adrenal axis in men with spinal cord injuries. Am J Phys Med Rehabil 1998;77:108–12.

[39] Shim HB, Jung TY, Lee JK, et al. Prostate activity and prostate cancer in spinal cord injury. Prostate Cancer Prostatic Dis 2006;9(2):115–20.

[40] De Marzo AM, Marchi VL, Epstein JI, et al. Proliferative inflammatory atrophy of the prostate: implications for prostatic carcinogenesis. Am J Pathol 1992;155:1985–92.

[41] Federman Q, Tannenbaum M, Vereczkey Z. Reduced incidence risk of prostatic carcinoma in patients with spinal cord injury. Am J Paraplegia 1993;16(Suppl):280.

[42] Scott PA Sr, Perkash I, Mode D, et al. Prostate cancer diagnosed in spinal cord-injured patients is more commonly advanced stage than in able-bodied patients. Urology 2004;63: 509–12.

[43] Wyndaele JJ, Iwatsubo E, Perkash I, et al. Prostate cancer: a hazard also to be considered in the ageing male patient with spinal cord injury. Spinal Cord 1998;36:299–302.

[44] Frisbie J, Chopra S, Foo D, et al. Colorectal carcinoma and myelopathy. J Am Paraplegia Soc 1984;7(2):33–6.

[45] Stratton MD, McKirgan LW, Wade TP, et al. Colorectal cancer in patients with previous spinal cord injury. Dis Colon Rectum 1996;39(9):965–8.

[46] Kirk PM, King RB, Temple R, et al. Long-term follow-up of bowel management after spinal cord injury. SCI Nurs 1997;14(2):56–63.

[47] Harvard report on cancer prevention. Vol. 1. Causes of human cancer. Cancer Causes Control 1996;7(Suppl 1):S3–9.

[48] Stiens SA, Bergman SB, Goetz LL. Neurogenic bowel dysfunction after spinal cord injury: clinical evaluation and rehabilitative management. Arch Phys Med Rehabil 1997;78(3 Suppl):S86–102.

[49] DeVivo MJ, Krause JS, Lammertse DP. Recent trends in mortality and causes of death among persons with spinal cord injury. Arch Phys Med Rehabil 1999;80(11):1411–9.

[50] Whiteneck GG, Charlifue SW, Frankel HL, et al. Mortality, morbidity, and psychosocial outcomes of persons spinal cord injured more than 20 years ago. Paraplegia 1992;30(9): 617–30.

[51] Department of Veterans Affairs. Fact sheet: VA and spinal cord injury. VA Office of Public Affairs. Available at: http://www.va.gov/pressrel/spinalcfs.htm. Accessed February 12, 2002.

[52] Brandon J. Health promotion and wellness in rehabilitation services. J Rehabil 1985;51(4): 54–8.

[53] Marge M. Health promotion for persons with disabilities: moving beyond rehabilitation. Am J Health Promot 1988;2:29–35.

[54] Warms CA. Health promotion services in post-rehabilitation spinal cord injury health care. Rehabil Nurs 1987;12:304–8.

[55] Burns TJ, Batavia AI, Smith QW, et al. Primary health care need of persons with physical disabilities: what are the research and service priorities? Arch Phys Med Rehabil 1990;71: 138–43.

[56] Menter RR, et al. Issues of aging with spinal cord injury. In: Whiteneck GG, Charlifue SW, Gerhart KA, editors. Aging with spinal cord injury. New York: Demos; 1993. p. 1–8.

[57] US Department of Health and Human Services. Healthy people 2010. Focus Area 6: Disability and secondary conditions. Available at: http://www.healthypeople.gov/Document/pdf/Volume1/06Disability.pdf. Accessed April 4, 2007.

[58] Centers for Disease Control and Prevention. Prevention of pneumococcal disease: Recommendations of the Advisory Committee on Immunization Practices (ACIP). MMWR Recomm Rep 1997;46(RR-8):1–25.

[59] U.S. Preventive Services Task Force. Screening for colorectal cancer: Recommendations and rationale. Rockville (MD): Agency for Healthcare Research and Quality; 2002. Available at: www.ahrq.gov/clinic/3rduspstf/colorectal/colorr.htm. Accessed January 4, 2007.
[60] Vickrey BG, Mittman BS, Connor KI, et al. The effect of a disease management intervention on quality and outcomes of dementia care: a randomized, controlled trial. Ann Intern Med 2006;145(10):713–26.
[61] Dean NC, Bateman KA, Donnelly SM, et al. Improving clinical outcomes with utilization of a community-acquired pneumonia guideline. Chest 2006;130(3):794–9.
[62] Sackett DL. Rules of evidence and clinical recommendations on the use of antithromobotic agents. Chest 1989;92(2 Suppl):2S–4S.
[63] Richardson WS. We should overcome the barriers to evidence-based clinical diagnosis! J Clin Epidemiol 2007;60(3):217–27.
[64] Paramonczyk A. Barriers to implementing research into clinical practice. Can Nurse 2005; 101(3):12–5.
[65] Wilmot CB, Hall KM, et al. The respiratory system. In: Whiteneck GG, Charlifue SW, Gerhart KA, editors. Aging with spinal cord injury. New York: Demos Publications; 1993. p. 93–104.
[66] National Spinal Injury Statistical Center. Annual Statistical Report for the Model Spinal Cord Injury Care System. University of Alabama, Birmingham 2005. Available at: http://images.main.uab.edu/spinalcord/pdffiles/factors05.pdf. Accessed January 4, 2007.
[67] Smith B, Weaver FM, LaVela SL, et al. Causes of death for veterans with spinal cord injuries and disorders. Presented at the HSR&D National Meeting, Department of Veterans Affairs. Arlington (VA), February 23, 2007.
[68] CDC. Public health and aging: Influenza vaccination coverage among adults aged $\geq$50 years and pneumococcal vaccination coverage among adults aged $\geq$65 years—United States, 2002. MMWR Morbid Mortal Wkly Rep 2003;52(4):987–92.
[69] CDC-ACIP. Prevention of pneumococcal disease: recommendations of the Advisory Committee on Immunization Practices (ACIP). MMWR Recomm Rep 1997;46(No. RR-8): 1–25.
[70] Nordin J, Mulloohy J, Poblete S, et al. Influenza vaccine effectiveness in preventing hospitalizations and deaths in persons 65 years or older in Minnesota. New York and Oregon: data from 3 health plans. J Infect Dis 2001;184:665–70.
[71] CDC-ACIP. Prevention and control of influenza: recommendations of the Advisory Committee on Immunization Practices (ACIP). MMWR Recomm Rep 2001;50(No. RR-4):1–46.
[72] Trautner BW, Atmar RL, Hulstrom A, et al. Inactivated influenza vaccination for people with spinal cord injury. Arch Phys Med Rehabil 2004;85(11):1886–9.
[73] Consortium for Spinal Cord Medicine (CSCM). Respiratory management following SCI. Clinical practice guidelines. Paralyzed Veterans of America, Washington, DC; 2005.
[74] Veterans Health Administration. Spinal cord injury study. Performance report, office of quality and performance, Washington, DC; 1999.
[75] Evans C, Legro M, Weaver FM, et al. Perceptions about influenza vaccinations among veterans with spinal cord injury. J Spinal Cord Med 2003;26(3):204–9.
[76] Weaver FM, Goldstein B, Evans C, et al. Increasing influenza vaccination rates in veterans with spinal cord injuries and disorders. J Spinal Cord Med 2003;26(3):210–8.
[77] Weaver FM, Smith B, LaVela SL, et al. A multi-strategy approach to increase influenza vaccinations in veterans with spinal cord injuries and disorders. J Spinal Cord Med 2007;30:10–9.
[78] Spinal Cord Injury Quality Enhancement Research Initiative. Annual report Health Services Research & Development, Department of Veterans Affairs; 2006.
[79] Fishburn MJ, Marino RJ, Ditunno JF. Atelectasis and pneumonia in acute spinal cord injury. Arch Phys Med Rehabil 1990;71:197–200.

[80] Jackson AB, Groomes TE. Incidence of respiratory complications following spinal cord injury. Arch Phys Med Rehabil 1994;75:270–5.
[81] Spungen AM, Dicpinigaitis PV, Almenoff PL, et al. Pulmonary obstruction in individuals with cervical spinal cord lesions unmasked by bronchodilators. Paraplegia 1993;31:404–7.
[82] Linn WS, Spungen AM, Gong H, et al. Smoking and obstructive lung dysfunction in persons with chronic spinal cord injury. JSCM 2003;26(1):28–35.
[83] Davies DS, McColl MA. Lifestyle risks for three disease outcomes in spinal cord injury. Clin Rehabil 2002;16(1):96–108.
[84] Kocina P. Body composition of spinal cord injured adults. Sports Med 1997;23(1):48–60.
[85] Centers for Disease Control. Cigarette smoking among adults- United States. Mortality and Morbidity Weekly Report 2005;55(54):1121–4.
[86] Weaver FM, LaVela SL, Miskevics S, et al. Smoking behavior and readiness to change in veterans with spinal cord injuries and disorders. Rehabil Psychol, in press.
[87] Jonk YC, Sherman SE, Fu SS, et al. National trends in the provision of smoking cessation aids within the Veterans Health Administration. Am J Manag Care 2005;11(2):77–85.
[88] Office of Quality Performance. Technical manual for FY2007. External peer review process. Office of quality and performance. Washington, DC: Veterans Health Administration; 2006.
[89] Williams-Slegle C, Ellwood M, Kennedy D, et al. Smoking cessation in a spinal cord injury population. Presented at the AASCIPSW Annual Meeting. Las Vegas (NV), September, 2004.
[90] Consortium for Spinal Cord Medicine (CSCM). Neurogenic bowel management in adults with spinal cord injury. Washington, DC: Paralyzed Veterans of America; 1998.
[91] Roach MH, Frost FS, Creasey G. Social and personal consequences of acquired bowel dysfunction for persons with spinal cord injury. J Spinal Cord Med 2000;23:263–9.
[92] Stiens SA, Fajardo NR, Korsten MA. The gastrointestinal system after spinal cord injury. In: Liv V, editor. Spinal cord medicine: principles and practice. New York: Demos Medical Publishing; 2003. p. 321–48.
[93] Goetz LL, Nelson AL, Guihan ML, et al. Provider adherence to implementation of clinical practice guidelines for neurogenic bowel in adults with spinal cord injury. J Spinal Cord Med 2005;28(5):394–406.

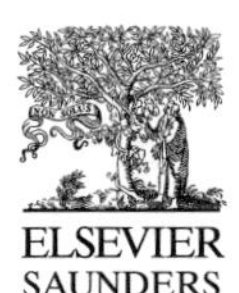

ELSEVIER
SAUNDERS

Phys Med Rehabil Clin N Am 18 (2007) 317–331

PHYSICAL MEDICINE AND REHABILITATION CLINICS OF NORTH AMERICA

Cardiovascular Health and Fitness in Persons with Spinal Cord Injury

Timothy D. Lavis, MD*, William M. Scelza, MD, William L. Bockenek, MD

Carolinas Rehabilitation, 1100 Blythe Blvd., Charlotte, NC 28203, USA

As both the number of people and life expectancy increase for people with spinal cord injuries (SCI), many health concerns related to aging start to play a significant role in their overall health. Estimates for the incidence of new SCI remain approximately 11,000 per year, and the prevalence is approximately 230,000 and growing [1]. Although life expectancies continue to rise with improved emergent and long-term management techniques, life expectancies remain below that of the general population [1]. The effects of aging with spinal cord injury also have become more prevalent with greater lifespans. Among SCI survivors in the United States, it is believed that 40% are older than 45 years, and about 1 in 4 has lived 20 years or longer with their SCI [2].

Coronary heart disease (CHD) remains the leading cause of mortality among all Americans accounting for nearly 500,000 deaths per year [3]. All individuals face numerous risk factors for CHD (Table 1) [4]. Individuals with SCI have been shown to be at increased risk of premature CHD development [5–8]. Epidemiologic studies have found heart disease to be the cause or contributing factor in 22.4% of all deaths among those with SCI [9]. In patients with chronic SCI, cardiovascular disease was the most frequent cause of death accounting for 46% of all deaths in people greater than 30 years after injury [10]. Groah and colleagues [11] has also shown that individuals with advancing age and higher levels and severity of SCI were at greater risk for CHD. Asymptomatic heart disease also has been detected among people with both tetraplegia and paraplegia, making early identification of risk factors, diagnosis, and primary prevention of CHD even more crucial [12,13].

* Corresponding author.
E-mail address: timothy.lavis@carolinashealthcare.org (T.D. Lavis).

1047-9651/07/$ - see front matter
doi:10.1016/j.pmr.2007.03.003

Table 1
Major risk factors for CHD

Modifiable risk factors	Nonmodifiable risk factors
Cigarette smoking	Age (men ≥45; women ≥55)
Hypertension	Family history
Low HDL-C[a] <40	
Diabetes	

[a] HDL cholesterol ≥60 counts as a negative risk factor equivalent.

Data from National Cholesterol Education Program (NCEP) Expert Panel on Detection. Third Report of the National Cholesterol Education Program (NCEP) Expert Panel on Detection, Evaluation, and Treatment of High Blood Cholesterol in Adults (Adult Treatment Panel III) final report. Circulation 2002;106(25):3143–421.

Several of the key cardiovascular risk factors have been shown to be more prevalent in individuals with SCI [6,8,14]. Changes in body composition and lower levels of physical activity in persons with SCI are significant contributors to this increased risk for cardiovascular disease. These include changes in lipid metabolism, glucose intolerance/diabetes, obesity, and lack of physical fitness.

Lipid metabolism

High-density lipoproteins (HDL) account for approximately 20% to 30% of total levels of serum cholesterol. The precise mechanisms involved in the protective effects of HDL have not been elucidated fully. Thoughts on its benefit include its action as an antioxidant, antiinflammatory agent, and an inhibitor of atherogenesis [4]. Studies have found a correlation with low levels of HDL and increased risk for the development of CHD. Conversely, elevated levels of serum HDL have shown protective effects. HDL levels <40 mg/dL are an independent risk factor for the development of CHD. Approximately 10% of the general population has HDL levels <35 mg/dL versus up to 40% in the SCI population [7,15,16]. Those with tetraplegia have been shown to have lower levels of HDL versus paraplegia, suggesting that decreased physical activity is a major contributor to lower HDL levels [6]. Increased levels of cardiopulmonary fitness have been shown to elevate levels of HDL in both the SCI and able-bodied populations [15,17,18].

Low-density lipoproteins (LDL) make up approximately 60% to 70% of serum cholesterol levels. It is believed to be the primary atherogenic cholesterol compound. Deposits of cholesterol, primarily LDL, originate in the coronary arteries and, over time, mature into occlusive plaques in the coronary arteries. Approximately 25% of the general population is considered to have elevated levels of LDL cholesterol. Individuals with SCI have been shown to have LDL levels similar to that of the general population [5]. Because of the positive association with LDL and the increased risk of

CHD, LDL is the primary target for lipid-lowering therapy, with the goal of treatment to lower serum LDL levels. Strategies such as low-fat, low-cholesterol dietary changes and increased physical activity often are first-line therapeutic strategies. Drugs such as the 5-hydroxy-3-methylglutaryl-coenzyme + A + reductase (HMG Co-A) reductase inhibitors may also be necessary when LDL levels are resistant to the lifestyle changes. These agents act in the liver to decrease the biosynthesis of LDL levels. Other agents such as bile acid sequestrants or resins can also be useful adjunct therapy in the management of hypercholesterolemia. Drug therapy is also predicated on the risk factor analysis of an individual. Those people with elevated LDL levels and two or more risk factors are treated much more aggressively with lipid-lowering medications and have lower target LDL values (Tables 2 and 3) [4]. Because individuals with SCI have an increased likelihood of having an increased number of risk factors (elevated HDL, obesity, altered glucose metabolism), aggressive monitoring of LDL levels are crucial.

Serum triglycerides are also thought to contribute to CHD. Although they are not identified as an independent risk factor for CHD, elevated levels of triglycerides are very commonly associated with some nonlipid risk factors for CHD including those with diabetes, obesity, high carbohydrate diets, sedentary lifestyles, hypertension, excess alcohol intake, and cigarette smoking [4]. Both individuals with SCI and able-bodied controls show an inverse correlation with HDL cholesterol (HDL-C) levels and triglyceride levels [15].

Glucose intolerance/diabetes

Abnormalities in glucose metabolism are also more prevalent in individuals with SCI [19,20]. After an SCI, atrophy of skeletal muscle decreases the muscle mass. It has been shown that by 24 weeks after injury the cross-sectional muscle mass of the leg is 45% to 80% of age-matched controls [21]. Subjects with tetraplegia have been found to have a reduction in glucose transport that is proportional to the loss of the muscle mass [21,22].

Table 2
Target for LDL-cholesterol (mg/dL)

<100	Optimal
100–129	Near optimal
130–159	Borderline
160–189	High
≥190	Very high

Data from National Cholesterol Education Program (NCEP) Expert Panel on Detection. Third Report of the National Cholesterol Education Program (NCEP) Expert Panel on Detection, Evaluation, and Treatment of High Blood Cholesterol in Adults (Adult Treatment Panel III) final report. Circulation 2002;106(25):3143–421.

Table 3
Risk category

CHD present or CHD risk >20%	<100
2+ risk factors (10-year risk ≤20%)	<130
0–1 risk factors	<160

Data from National Cholesterol Education Program (NCEP) Expert Panel on Detection. Third Report of the National Cholesterol Education Program (NCEP) Expert Panel on Detection, Evaluation, and Treatment of High Blood Cholesterol in Adults (Adult Treatment Panel III) final report. Circulation 2002;106(25):3143–421.

The loss of muscle mass is critical because insulin acts peripherally on the individual's muscle mass for metabolism of glucose. Glucose tolerance ensues as higher plasma levels of insulin are required to maintain normal blood glucose levels [23]. Elevated serum insulin levels and other abnormalities in glucose metabolism, even if not meeting criteria for absolute diabetes, are considered to be atherogenic conditions, increasing the risk for CHD.

Bauman and colleagues [20] have shown the increased rates of abnormal glucose tolerance and presence of frank diabetes in individuals with SCI compared with age-matched controls. After a 75-g oral glucose tolerance test, 22% of individuals with SCI had met criteria for diabetes versus only 6% of the able-bodied subjects tested. Only 38% of individuals with tetraplegia and 50% of those with paraplegia had a normal response to this glucose tolerance test versus 82% of age-matched controls. Bauman [20] also found that those with complete tetraplegia were found to have the highest incidence of impaired glucose metabolism compared with other neurologic classification groups of spinal cord injury, stressing the importance of muscle mass and immobility.

Obesity

Obesity is also a major risk factor contributing to increased risk of CHD in the population with SCI. Obesity after SCI can come about from a number of factors. Buchholz [24] estimates that the resting metabolic rate (RMR) is overestimated by 5% to 32% in individuals with SCI. This is explained primarily by a reduction in the fat-free lean body mass. In normal individuals, the RMR typically will account for approximately 65% of the total energy expenditure. After SCI, there is a decrease in the fat-free body mass that occurs primarily from atrophy of skeletal muscle. Studies have shown that the RMR has been found to be 14% to 27% lower in individuals with chronic SCI versus age-matched control subjects [24,25]. Absence of this metabolically active muscle can account for a significant portion of the decreased resting metabolic rate. It is also thought in high-level injuries that the decreased sympathetic nervous system activity can contribute to a decreased RMR. The issue of obesity in people with SCI is extensively reviewed by Dr. Gater in this edition of *PM&R clinics*.

Physical fitness

Physical activity accounts for 25% to 30% of the total daily energy expenditure [26]. Not surprisingly, numerous studies suggest that individuals with SCI have significantly lower levels of regular physical activity than the able-bodied population [27]. It is also noted that individuals with tetraplegia had lower levels of fitness versus those with paraplegia [28–30]. The thermal effect of food accounts for approximately 10% of the total daily energy expenditure and is not felt to be significantly different in the able-bodied population versus the population with SCI. This decrease in RMR and decreased physical activity in individuals with SCI can lead to a positive energy balance. Individuals with SCI have been found to have lower metabolic demands and decreased energy expenditures. To maintain weight at baseline levels, caloric intake must be reduced accordingly or weight gain will occur [26].

Individuals with SCI, by the nature of their impairments, are susceptible to the constellation of metabolic abnormalities discussed above (decreased HDL-C levels, glucose intolerance/insulin resistance, type II diabetes mellitus, obesity, and sedentary lifestyle). This cluster of clinical and subclinical metabolic risk factors, the metabolic syndrome, has been associated with increased risk for CHD [31]. Regular physical activity can increase exercise capacity, endurance, and muscle strength and has clearly been associated with decreased risk of cardiovascular disease. High levels of exercise have shown positive effects on lipoprotein profiles [18]. Meta-analysis of 52 exercise trials of exercise training programs of > 12 weeks' duration yielded significant increases of HDL-C and decreases in both LDL cholesterol (LDL-C) and triglycerides [32]. The HEalth, RIsk factors, exercise Training, And GEnetics (HERITAGE) study, a large and carefully controlled exercise study, also found positive effects on HDL-C, triglycerides, and LDL-C levels [33].

Physical activity has also shown positive effects on glucose metabolism [17]. A diabetes prevention program showed that with an 8–metabolic equivalent (MET)-hour/week increase of activity (roughly equivalent to 6 miles of walking per week) showed a 58% decrease in the onset of type II diabetes and an average of a 4-kg weight loss compared with usual management [34]. A review of 337 patients with type II diabetes showed average reductions in hemoglobin A1c levels of 0.5% to 1.0% [35].

Exercise alone is an inefficient means to achieve weight loss, and programs incorporating both an increase in physical activity and lifestyle modification produce better results [36,37]. Exercise is certainly an important component in the battle with obesity. Exercise assists in fat metabolism and gains in lean muscle mass that can very well improve the general body composition [38]. In contrast, weight loss programs with dieting can contribute to a 30% loss in lean muscle mass. A loss in weight of 5% to 10% can produce improvements in other cardiovascular risk factors [36]. In general, the benefits of increased physical activity have widely been defined as an important component to a wellness program.

The American College of Sports Medicine (ACSM) and Centers for Disease Control (CDC) recommend that healthy adults participate in 30 minutes or more of moderate-intensity physical activity (ie, brisk walking) on most, and preferably all, days of the week [17]. Moderate intensity exercises are classified as 40% to 60% of one's peak VO_2 max or 4 to 6 metabolic equivalents (METs). One MET (3.5 mL O_2/kg/min) is equivalent to one's energy expenditure at total rest. A brisk walk of about 3 miles per hour is roughly equivalent to 4 METs [17]. Evidence shows that exercise can also decrease the risks of other chronic diseases such as type II diabetes mellitus and obesity [35,38].

Sedentary lifestyles and decreased amounts of physical activity, however, are common among individuals with and without SCI. One survey estimates that more than 60% of Americans reported infrequent activity and one of four people stated they were totally sedentary [39]. Individuals with SCI are perhaps even more susceptible to the perils of a sedentary lifestyle as a direct result of there injury and limited options for exercise [27]. Studies suggest that those with SCI have significantly lower levels of physical activity than those in the able-bodied population [40]. In fact, individuals living with SCI have been placed in the low end of the physical fitness spectrum. As expected, individuals with tetraplegia have lower levels of daily energy expenditure and aerobic power than those with paraplegia [41,42]. Those with paraplegia, despite their increased upper extremity mobility and options for exercise, have been found to be only marginally more fit than those with tetraplegia [43]. Noreau and colleagues [27] has shown that approximately 25% of young people with paraplegia were able to achieve peak oxygen consumption levels that were only marginally sufficient to maintain independent living.

In an effort to combat many of the secondary conditions that occur after spinal cord injury, regular exercise and active lifestyles should be encouraged for all people with spinal cord injuries. The options for activity and types of exercise available vary depending on local resources, interests, and accessibility. In addition to the physical and metabolic benefits of exercise, persons with spinal cord injury who exercised reported less stress, less depression, and an improved quality of life [44]. With regard to exercising after spinal cord injury, there are several physiologic changes that occur that have significant effect on exercise response and tolerance. These include the impairment or loss of sensorimotor function below the neurologic level of injury and impairments of the autonomic nervous system.

After spinal cord injury, there is loss of voluntary motor function in the large muscle groups in the lower extremities. This loss generally limits exercise routines to the smaller muscle groups of the upper extremities and trunk. The overall availability of muscle mass is dependent on level and completeness of injury and varies between individuals. An inverse relationship between level of injury and the peak oxygen consumption and cardiac output has been observed during exercise in those with spinal cord injury [45,46]. Individuals with paraplegia have peak power output and cardiac output levels approximately half of those on able-bodied persons performing lower extremity exercise [46]. The levels in tetraplegia are even further reduced from those seen with paraplegia [45]. As the level of injury increases, less muscle mass is available during exercise. During peak exercise, individuals with higher-level lesions may have more difficulty reaching levels of O_2 consumption that stress the cardiovascular system appropriately before they reach peripheral fatigue. Persons with tetraplegia may also be less efficient during exercise because of the loss of trunk control and the need to stabilize themselves with the same muscle groups they are attempting to exercise [47].

In the able-bodied population, during exercise, there is a physiologic response that accounts for appropriate flow and distribution of blood throughout the body. This is accomplished with the venous pumping action of the lower extremities as well as through sympathetic-mediated input to maintain systemic blood pressure and flow. This ultimately allows for an increase in the cardiac end-diastolic volume, which increases the stroke volume of the heart and ultimately the cardiac output. This effect allows for greater delivery of oxygenated blood to the active muscles and compensation for their increased metabolic rate. In a person with spinal cord injury, this response can be significantly impaired. After spinal cord injury, in addition to the loss of lower extremity muscle activation during exercise, there are significant alterations in the flow and distribution of blood throughout the cardiovascular system. This results from loss of the venous pumping action in the muscles of the lower extremities as well as alterations in the autonomic (particularly sympathetic) nervous system that affects the cardiovascular system's response to exercise. Persons with higher-level thoracic and cervical injuries, in addition to impaired function and blood flow in the lower extremities, also may experience a partial or complete separation of the autonomic nervous system from central control. This autonomic dysfunction further affects the cardiac response to exercise and ultimately may lead to further impairment in peak cardiac output achieved during exercise.

Impaired blood flow caused by the loss of venous pumping action and compensatory vasoconstriction can lead to blood pooling in the lower extremities, which results in decreased stroke volume both at rest and during exercise. Impairment in stroke volume has a direct effect on the resulting cardiac output. Several techniques have been evaluated to decrease the blood pooling in the lower extremities and improve blood return to the heart. These techniques include arm crank exercise in the supine or leg-elevated position, lower extremity compression garments, abdominal binders, antigravity suits (increase external pressure on the lower extremities), and lower extremity functional electrical stimulation (FES) [48].

Hopman and colleagues [48], conducted a comprehensive study comparing submaximal arm crank exercise response in tetraplegia and paraplegia using several different techniques to improve blood flow and redistribution. When compared with submaximal exercise in the sitting position, this study showed varied responses depending on the technique used. Supine positioning resulted in decreased heart rate and increased stroke volume significantly in both groups. The antigravity suit decreased heart rate in both groups and decreased oxygen uptake in those with paraplegia. Compressive stockings decreased heart rate and increased stroke volume in those with paraplegia only. FES improved stroke volume and increased oxygen uptake in the group with tetraplegia. This finding showed that the benefits of different techniques vary depending on mechanism and level of spinal cord injury [48].

In addition to the mechanical effects of lower-extremity paralysis and the affect it has on blood flow, the autonomic dysfunction following spinal cord injury also has a significant influence on exercise response. This dysfunction leads to alterations in heart rate, stroke volume, cardiac output, and blood pressure when compared with able-bodied controls [49]. The sympathetic output from the spinal cord occurs from the T1 through the L2 level, and autonomic function and the body's response may vary depending on the exact neurologic level and completeness of injury. In persons with tetraplegia, where injury occurs above sympathetic output of the spinal cord, there is a separation of the central control for autonomic nervous system from the periphery. Persons with tetraplegia typically have resting hypotensive blood pressures with systolic pressures in the 70- to 80-mmHg range when in the sitting position. The autonomic impairment affects the central control over input to the heart, adrenals, and peripheral vascular system [50]. At maximal exercise effort, the peak heart rate seen with tetraplegia is generally limited to approximately 120 to 130 beats per minute. It has been suggested that this is most likely regulated through a decrease in parasympathetic input without sympathetic compensation [50]. During exercise, sympathetic impairment also leads to loss of the sympathetic-mediated vasoconstriction used to regulate blood flow in the muscles and skin with the end result being the inability to maintain systemic blood pressure and thermoregulation; this may result in uncompensated vasodilation, with further hypotension and dizziness during more strenuous exercise. The long-term effects of low systemic blood pressure and impaired cardiac preload eventually can result in myocardium atrophy and impaired cardiac efficiency [51].

In studies of persons with paraplegia with injury levels T1 through T4, sympathetic input and exercise response have shown inconclusive results [52]. Approaching levels of T6 and below, there is generally sustained central control of sympathetic regulation. Individuals with mid-level thoracic lesions and below are able to maintain normotensive blood pressures and cardiac output levels similar to able-bodied controls at rest. The sympathetic cardiac response allows for these individuals to compensate for decreased stroke volume secondary to the venous pooling in the lower extremities by elevating the heart rate, which is not seen in tetraplegia. Therefore, to maintain a similar cardiac output as able-bodied persons in the face of a lower stroke volume, resting heart rates are generally higher in those with lesions below T5 than in those in the uninjured population. Heart rates in paraplegia patients are also higher at similar workloads during exercise [52]. The overall effect of heart rate on cardiac output is somewhat limited in paraplegia, and elevation of heart rate is unable to fully compensate adequately to increase the cardiac output to a level similar to able-bodied controls during more rigorous exercise using the upper extremities [53].

Even in the presence of the changes in exercise response, benefits to exercise have been defined clearly in individuals with SCI. In studies that have examined the relationship of peak oxygen consumption (VO_2 max) obtained via arm ergometry and serum lipids, significant inverse relationships were found between the VO_2 max and total cholesterol to HDL-C ratios, triglycerides, and LDL-C to HDL-C ratio [43]. High-intensity training also showed increased levels of HDL-C and decreased triglycerides, LDL-C, and total cholesterol to HDL C ratios [54]. Exercise testing of 22 men with paraplegia found that those with lower peak aerobic capacities (based on exercise testing) and lower physical activity levels had higher fasting glucose levels, decreased HDL-C levels, and larger abdominal girth [55]. With regard to cardiovascular improvements, in a review of 13 exercise studies, Hoffmann [56] noted VO_2 max improvements after several weeks of training. In a study evaluating benefits of a 12-week circuit training program for person with paraplegia, Jacobs and colleagues [57], observed increased peak oxygen consumption, time to fatigue, peak power output, and improved isoinertial and isokinetic strength. Many of the benefits resulting from arm exercise routines are felt to be peripheral in nature or resulting more from changes in the arm musculature that leads to improvements in strength and endurance rather than from cardiovascular adaptations.

In addition to arm exercise, FES leg cycle ergometry (FES-LCE) also has been evaluated for its potential to activate lower-extremity muscles and improve blood flow back to the heart where it could improve stroke volume and cardiac output [58,59]. In a 12- to 16-week study involving 36 exercise sessions in which persons with both tetraplegia and paraplegia performed FES-LCE, Hooker and colleagues [58] observed higher posttraining power output, oxygen uptake, pulmonary ventilation, heart rate and cardiac output, and lower total peripheral resistance. In another study involving FES-LCE over 12 weeks with 36 sessions, Faghri and colleagues [59] observed increased power output, in both tetraplegia and paraplegia. He also noted increased resting heart rate and systolic blood pressure in the group with tetraplegia, suggesting better cardiovascular stability. In both groups, heart rate and blood pressure decreased while stroke volume and cardiac output increased after 12 weeks. Exercise programs with

FES-LCE also have been reported to reverse the left ventricular myocardial atrophy seen with tetraplegia [60].

The need for exercise in the SCI population has been well recognized and does not vary dramatically from the general population. Generally, it is suggested that three to five exercise sessions should occur on a weekly basis. These sessions should be 20 to 60 minutes in duration with an intensity of 50% to 80% of the individual's peak heart rate [61]. The American College of Sports medicine has published recommended exercise programming for individuals with SCI [61]. The recommendations for these exercise programs are summarized as follows: different modes of cardiopulmonary training, which includes arm crank ergometry, wheelchair propulsion, swimming, vigorous wheelchair sports, ambulation with crutches or braces, seated aerobic exercise, and the use of electrically stimulated leg cycle activities. Important considerations in the prevention of overuse injuries are important components. It is suggested to try to vary activities as much as possible to avoid overuse injuries to the upper extremities as well as to provide strengthening activities to all major muscle groups. Emphasis on precautions, to minimize the risk of secondary conditions that individuals with SCI are susceptible to are also emphasized. Using appropriate pressure relief cushions and proper positioning and balancing to avoid falls and risk of fractures are outlined. In addition, autonomic dysfunction and autonomic dysreflexia are addressed, and it is suggested that consultation with a physician should occur if there are any questions regarding potential complications or secondary conditions. Slow, progressive improvements should be the goal, and expectations should be based on the amount of the muscle mass being exercised (ie, the greater the muscle mass being exercised, the greater the improvements in fitness that would be expected).

Barriers to exercise

Despite these defined problems associated with sedentary lifestyles after SCI (ie, depressed levels of HDL-C, glucose intolerance or diabetes, obesity) and the defined benefits of exercise after SCI, significant physical and psychological barriers to physical activity still exist. Healthy People 2010 suggested that individuals with disabilities were more likely to encounter problematic barriers than those in the able-bodied population [62]. In a study to evaluate the perceived barriers to exercise that individuals with SCI face, participants identified poor accessibility, lack of privacy, fear of injury, and public exposure of their injuries as major concerns to engaging in an exercise program [29]. Participants also identified lack of experience among staff at fitness centers in dealing with persons with SCI as a problem when starting an exercise routine [29]. Facilities that provide accessible environments are very limited and have also been noted as a common physical barrier [29]. Cardinal and colleagues [63] found that only 8% of fitness facilities provided adequate accessibility around actual exercise equipment, making it difficult for individuals who use wheelchairs to safely access the equipment. Sallis and colleagues [64] also described that in the general population, a lack of social support, unavailability of facilities, time constraints, and cost were main barriers to physical activity programs. Compared with the general population, individuals with SCI have similarly low motivation levels, and this remains one of the largest barriers to starting and maintaining an exercise program. Motivation and exercise self-efficacy were more powerful predictors of exercise maintenance in individuals with disabilities than disability-related characteristics or environmental barriers [65].

There remains a need for exercise opportunities that are tailored to the issues faced by individuals with SCI, such as the need for accessible facilities and equipment [29]. Among the most obvious barriers to full participation are architectural barriers and adaptive equipment. Cardinal and colleagues report that 92% of fitness facilities failed to provide adequate accessibility around exercise equipment. Perceived barriers to exercise are also potential deterrents. In a recent study among individuals with SCI, lack of privacy, fear of injury, lack of professional training and limited clinical experience among staff, and public exposure of their injury were identified as deterrents to engaging in an exercise program [29].

Surprisingly little is known about the factors that determine adherence to community-based exercise programs. One study has suggested that use of a personal trainer did improve exercise program attendance but had little effect on overall weight loss [66]. The investigators did not evaluate the motivation of the subjects that actually participated in the program, but they only studied the effects of adding a trainer. Results from another study of previously sedentary women were more encouraging [67]. Subjects were enrolled in a structured and supervised exercise program and transitioned to a home program. They were also provided with practical sessions on how to properly prepare and engage in exercise. This study did show that a center-based and closely supervised exercise program results in both short- and long-term exercise retention rates [67]. In another study testing individuals with SCI, Hicks and colleagues [44] showed, in a structured twice-weekly exercise program, improved muscle strength, ergometry performance, and quality of life in individuals who completed the program. Follow-up on the maintenance of these individuals showed significant dropout after 3 months [63]. Individuals in this study were never presented with a comprehensive approach to wellness, and the interactions were limited to twice a week, an intensity that is hardly adequate for this population. Although the investigators do not specify, social interactions and the opportunity to network with peers would appear to be important factors.

We should be cautious when generalizing comparisons from studies with able-bodied individuals to those with SCI. Unlike able-bodied individuals, persons with a SCI are unique in their needs. As outlined above, people with SCI face numerous physical and psychological barriers to exercise that able-bodied individuals do not face, and it is recommended that individuals with SCI have appropriate assistance with positioning and placement when using equipment and may require motivational techniques that extend beyond those for the people without disabilities. Exercise professionals who receive specialized training and hands-on clinical experience before working with persons with SCI will be more adept to provide psychological as well as physical support, which we believe will maximize adherence to such programs [61,68].

References

[1] National Spinal Cord Injury Statistical Center. Spinal cord injury. Facts and figures at a glance. J Spinal Cord Med 2005;28(4):379–80.

[2] Gerhart KA, Bergstrom E, Charlifue SW, et al. Long-term spinal cord injury: functional changes over time. Arch Phys Med Rehabil 1993;74(10):1030–4.

[3] Thom T, Haase N, Rosamond W, et al. Heart disease and stroke statistics–2006 update: a report from the American Heart Association Statistics Committee and Stroke Statistics Subcommittee. Circulation 2006;113(6):e85–151.

[4] National Cholesterol Education Program (NCEP) Expert Panel on Detection EaToHBCiAATPI. Third Report of the National Cholesterol Education Program (NCEP) Expert Panel on Detection, Evaluation, and Treatment of High Blood Cholesterol in Adults (Adult Treatment Panel III) final report [see comment]. Circulation 2002;106(25): 314–421.

[5] Bauman WA, Kahn NN, Grimm DR, et al. Risk factors for atherogenesis and cardiovascular autonomic function in persons with spinal cord injury [review] [191 refs]. Spinal Cord 1999;37(9):601–16.

[6] Bauman WA, Adkins RH, Spungen AM, et al. The effect of residual neurological deficit on serum lipoproteins in individuals with chronic spinal cord injury. Spinal Cord 1998;36(1): 13–7.

[7] Brenes G, Dearwater S, Shapera R, et al. High density lipoprotein cholesterol concentrations in physically active and sedentary spinal cord injured patients. Arch Phys Med Rehabil 1986; 67(7):445–50.

[8] Yekutiel M, Brooks ME, Ohry A, et al. The prevalence of hypertension, ischaemic heart disease and diabetes in traumatic spinal cord injured patients and amputees. Paraplegia 1989;27(1):58–62.

[9] DeVivo MJ, Kartus PL, Stover SL, et al. Cause of death for patients with spinal cord injuries. Arch Intern Med 1989;149(8):1761–6.

[10] Whiteneck GG, Charlifue SW, Frankel HL, et al. Mortality, morbidity, and psychosocial outcomes of persons spinal cord injured more than 20 years ago. Paraplegia 1992;30(9): 617–30.

[11] Groah SL, Weitzenkamp D, Sett P, et al. The relationship between neurological level of injury and symptomatic cardiovascular disease risk in the aging spinal injured. Spinal Cord 2001;39(6):310–7.

[12] Bauman WA, Raza M, Chayes Z, et al. Tomographic thallium-201 myocardial perfusion imaging after intravenous dipyridamole in asymptomatic subjects with quadriplegia. Arch Phys Med Rehabil 1993;74(7):740–4.

[13] Bauman WA, Raza M, Spungen AM, et al. Cardiac stress testing with thallium-201 imaging reveals silent ischemia in individuals with paraplegia. Arch Phys Med Rehabil 1994;75(9): 946–50.

[14] Demirel S, Demirel G, Tukek T, et al. Risk factors for coronary heart disease in patients with spinal cord injury in Turkey. Spinal Cord 2001;39(3):134–8.

[15] Bauman WA, Spungen AM, Zhong YG, et al. Depressed serum high density lipoprotein cholesterol levels in veterans with spinal cord injury. Paraplegia 1992;30(10):697–703.
[16] Bauman WA, Adkins RH, Spungen AM, et al. Is immobilization associated with an abnormal lipoprotein profile? Observations from a diverse cohort. Spinal Cord 1999;37(7):485–93.
[17] Thompson PD, Thompson PD. Exercise and physical activity in the prevention and treatment of atherosclerotic cardiovascular disease. Arterioscler Thromb Vasc Biol 2003; 23(8):1319–21.
[18] Kraus WE, Houmard JA, Duscha BD, et al. Effects of the amount and intensity of exercise on plasma lipoproteins [see comment]. N Engl J Med 2002;347(19):1483–92.
[19] Bauman WA, Spungen AM. Carbohydrate and lipid metabolism in chronic spinal cord injury [review] [126 refs]. J Spinal Cord Med 2001;24(4):266–77.
[20] Bauman WA, Spungen AM. Disorders of carbohydrate and lipid metabolism in veterans with paraplegia or quadriplegia: a model of premature aging. Metab Clin Exp 1994;43(6): 749–56.
[21] Castro MJ, Apple DF Jr, Hillegass EA, et al. Influence of complete spinal cord injury on skeletal muscle cross-sectional area within the first 6 months of injury. Eur J Appl Physiol Occup Physiol 1999;80(4):373–8.
[22] Bauman WA, Spungen AM. Body composition in aging: adverse changes in able-bodied persons and those with spinal cord injury. Top Spinal Cord Inj Rehabil 2001;6:22–36.
[23] Aksnes AK, Hjeltnes N, Wahlstrom EO, et al. Intact glucose transport in morphologically altered denervated skeletal muscle from quadriplegic patients. Am J Physiol 1996;271(3 Pt 1): E593–600.
[24] Buchholz AC, McGillivray CF, Pencharz PB. Differences in resting metabolic rate between paraplegic and able-bodied subjects are explained by differences in body composition. Am J Clin Nutr 2003;77(2):371–8.
[25] Jeon JY, Steadward RD, Wheeler GD, et al. Intact sympathetic nervous system is required for leptin effects on resting metabolic rate in people with spinal cord injury. J Clin Endocrinol Metab 2003;88(1):402–7.
[26] Buchholz AC, Pencharz PB. Energy expenditure in chronic spinal cord injury [review] [50 refs]. Curr Opin Clin Nutr Metab Care 2004;7(6):635–9.
[27] Noreau L, Shephard RJ, Simard C, et al. Relationship of impairment and functional ability to habitual activity and fitness following spinal cord injury. Int J Rehabil Res 1993;16(4): 265–75.
[28] Burkett LN, Chisum J, Stone W, et al. Exercise capacity of untrained spinal cord injured individuals and the relationship of peak oxygen uptake to level of injury. Paraplegia 1990; 28(8):512–21.
[29] Scelza WM, Kalpakjian CZ, Zemper ED, et al. Perceived barriers to exercise in people with spinal cord injury. Am J Phys Med Rehabil 2005;84(8):576–83.
[30] Figoni SF. Perspectives on cardiovascular fitness and SCI [erratum appears in J Am Paraplegia Soc 1991 Jan;14(1):21] [review] [89 refs]. J Am Paraplegia Soc 1990;13(4):63–71.
[31] Stone NJ. Focus on lifestyle change and the metabolic syndrome [review] [52 refs]. Endocrinol Metab Clin North Am 2004;33(3):493–508.
[32] Leon AS, Sanchez OA, Leon AS, et al. Response of blood lipids to exercise training alone or combined with dietary intervention [review] [86 refs]. Med Sci Sports Exerc 2001;33(Suppl 6): S502–15.
[33] Leon AS, Rice T, Mandel S, et al. Blood lipid response to 20 weeks of supervised exercise in a large biracial population: the HERITAGE family study. Metab Clin Exper 2000;49(4): 513–20.
[34] Knowler WC, Barret-Connor E, Fowler FE, et al. Diabetes Prevention Program Research Group. Reduction in the incidence of type 2 diabetes with lifestyle intervention or metformin. N Engl J Med 2002;346:393–403.
[35] Thompson PD, Crouse SF, Goodpaster B, et al. The acute versus the chronic response to exercise [review] [71 refs]. Med Sci Sports Exerc 2001;33(Suppl 6):S438–45.

[36] Executive summary of the clinical guidelines on the identification, evaluation, and treatment of overweight and obesity in adults [review] [4 refs]. Arch Intern Med 1998;158(17):1855–67.

[37] Wing RR, Wing RR. Physical activity in the treatment of the adulthood overweight and obesity: current evidence and research issues. Med Sci Sports Exerc 1999;31(Suppl 11): S547–52.

[38] Bensimhon DR, Kraus WE, Donahue MP. Obesity and physical activity: a review [review] [57 refs]. Am Heart J 2006;151(3):598–603.

[39] Surgeon General's report on physical activity and health. From the Centers for Disease Control and Prevention. JAMA 1996;276(7):522.

[40] Dearwater SR, LaPorte RE, Robertson RJ, et al. Activity in the spinal cord-injured patient: an epidemiologic analysis of metabolic parameters. Med Sci Sports Exerc 1986;18 (5):541–4.

[41] Gass GC, Watson J, Camp EM, et al. The effects of physical training on high level spinal lesion patients. Scand J Rehabil Med 1980;12(2):61–5.

[42] Figoni SF. Exercise responses and quadriplegia [review] [87 refs]. Med Sci Sports Exerc 1993; 25(4):433–41.

[43] Bostom AG, Toner MM, McArdle WD, et al. Lipid and lipoprotein profiles relate to peak aerobic power in spinal cord injured men. Med Sci Sports Exerc 1991;23(4):409–14.

[44] Hicks AL, Martin KA, Ditor DS, et al. Long-term exercise training in persons with spinal cord injury: effects on strength, arm ergometry performance and psychological well-being. Spinal Cord 2003;41(1):34–43.

[45] Van Loan MD, McCluer S, Loftin JM, et al. Comparison of physiological responses to maximal arm exercises among able-bodied, paraplegics and quadriplegics. Paraplegia 1987;25:397–405.

[46] Figoni SF. Exercise responses and paraplegia. Med Sci Sports Exerc 1993;25(4):433–41.

[47] Jacobs PL, Nash MS. Exercise recommendations for individuals with spinal cord injury [review] [282 refs]. Sports Med 2004;34(11):727–51.

[48] Hopman MTE, Monroe M, Dueck C, et al. Blood redistribution and circulatory responses to submaximal arm exercises in persons with spinal cord injury. Scand J Rehabil Med 1998;30: 167–75.

[49] Dela F, Mohr T, Jensen CM, et al. Cardiovascular control during exercise: insights from spinal cord-injured humans. Circulation 2003;107(16):2127–33.

[50] Takahashi M, Sakaguchi A, Matsukawa K, et al. Cardiovascular control during voluntary static exercise in humans with tetraplegia. J Appl Physiol 2004;97:2077–82.

[51] Kessler KM, Pina I, Green B, et al. Cardiovascular findings in quadriplegic and paraplegic patients and in normal subjects. Am J Cardiol 1986;58(252):525–30.

[52] Schmid A, Huonker M, Barturen JM, et al. Catecholamines, heart rate and oxygen uptake during exercise in persons with spinal cord injury. J Appl Physiol 1998;85: 635–41.

[53] Jacobs PL, Mahoney ET, Robbins A, et al. Hypokinetic circulation in persons with paraplegia. Med Sci Sports Exerc 2002;34(9):1401–7.

[54] Hooker SP, Wells CL. Physiologic responses of elite paraplegic road racers to prolonged exercise. J Am Paraplegia Soc 1990;13(4):72–7.

[55] Manns PJ, McCubbin JA, Williams DP. Fitness, inflammation, and the metabolic syndrome in men with paraplegia. Arch Phys Med Rehabil 2005;86(6):1176–81.

[56] Hoffman M. Cardiorespiratory fitness and training in quadriplegics and paraplegics. Sports Med 1986;3:312–30.

[57] Jacobs PL, Nash MS, Rusinowski JW. Circuit training provides cardiorespiratory and strength benefits in persons with paraplegia. Med Sci Sports Exerc 2001;33(5): 711–7.

[58] Hooker S, Figoni S, Rodgers M, et al. Physiologic effects on electrical stimulation leg cycle exercise training in spinal cord injured persons. Arch Phys Med Rehabil 1992;73: 470–6.

[59] Faghri P, Glaser R, Figoni S. Functional electrical stimulation leg cycle ergometer exercise: the training effects on cardiorespiratory responses of spinal cord injured subjects at rest and during submaximal exercise. Arch Phys Med Rehabil 1992;73:1085–93.

[60] Nash MS, Bilskere S, Marcillo AE, et al. Reversal of adaptive left ventricular atrophy following electrically stimulated exercise training in human tetraplegics. Paraplegia 1991; 29:590–1.

[61] Figoni SF. Spinal cord disabilities: paraplegia and tetraplegia. In: Durstine JL, Moore GE, editors. ACSM's exercise management for persons with chronic diseases and disabilities. Champaign, IL: Human Kinetics; 2003. p. 247–53.

[62] U.S. Department of Health and Human Services. Office of Disease Prevention and Health Promotion–Healthy People 2010. Nasnewsletter 2000;15(3):3.

[63] Cardinal BJ, Kosma M, McCubbin JA. Factors influencing the exercise behavior of adults with physical disabilities. Med Sci Sports Exerc 2004;36(5):868–75.

[64] Sallis JF, Hovell MF, Hofstetter CR, et al. Predictors of adoption and maintenance of vigorous physical activity in men and women. Prev Med 1992;21(2):237–51.

[65] Kinne S, Patrick DL, Maher EJ, et al. Correlates of exercise maintenance among people with mobility impairments. Disability & Rehabilitation 1999;21(1):15–22.

[66] Jeffery RW, Wing RR, Thorson C, et al. Use of personal trainers and financial incentives to increase exercise in a behavioral weight-loss program. J Consult Clin Psychol 1998;66(5): 777–83.

[67] Cox KL, Burke V, Gorely TJ, et al. Controlled comparison of retention and adherence in home- vs center-initiated exercise interventions in women ages 40-65 years: The S.W.E.A.T. Study (Sedentary Women Exercise Adherence Trial). Prev Med 2003;36(1): 17–29.

[68] Figoni SF, Kiratli BJ, Sasaki R. Spinal cord dysfunction. In: Darcy PJ, editor. ACSM's resources for clinical exercise physiology: musculoskeletal, neuromuscular, neoplastic, immunologic, and hematologic conditions. Philadelphia, PA: Lippincott Williams & Wilkins; 2002. p. 48–67.

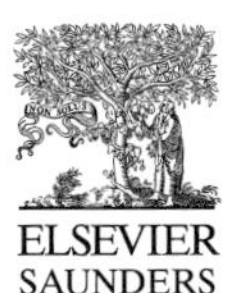

ELSEVIER
SAUNDERS

Phys Med Rehabil Clin N Am
18 (2007) 333–351

PHYSICAL MEDICINE
AND REHABILITATION
CLINICS OF
NORTH AMERICA

Obesity After Spinal Cord Injury

David R. Gater, Jr, MD, PhD[a,b,*]

[a] *Spinal Cord Injury and Disorders Center, Hunter Holmes McGuire VAMC (652/128), 1201 Broad Rock Boulevard, Richmond, VA 23249, USA*

[b] *Department of Physical Medicine and Rehabilitation, Virginia Commonwealth University, 1223 East Marshall Street, Richmond, VA 23298-0677, USA*

America is in the midst of an obesity epidemic, and individuals who have spinal cord injury (SCI) are perhaps at greater risk than any other segment of the population. Recent changes in the way obesity has been defined have lulled SCI practitioners into a false sense of security about the health of their patients regarding the dangers of obesity and its sequelae. This article defines and uses a definition of obesity that is more relevant to persons who have SCI, reviews the physiology of adipose tissue, and discusses aspects of heredity and environment that contribute to obesity in SCI. The pathophysiology of obesity is discussed relative to health risks for persons who have SCI, particularly those contributing to cardiovascular disease. Prevalence of obesity and its comorbidities are discussed and management options reviewed.

Definitions

"Obesity is a chronic, relapsing, neurochemical disease produced by the interaction of environment and host" [1]. In the late 1970s and 1980s, health researchers began to report an association between body fat and cardiovascular disease comorbidities, including hypertension, hyperlipidemia, and diabetes. Obesity was defined as an accumulation of excess body fat, with thresholds associated with cardiovascular disease greater than 22% body fat (%BF) for men and greater than 35% for women.

* Chief, Spinal Cord Injury and Disease, Department of Veterans Affairs, Hunter Holmes McGuire Medical Center, Spinal Cord Injury and Disorders Service (652/128), 1201 Broad Rock Boulevard, Richmond, VA 23249.

E-mail address: David.Gater@va.gov

1047-9651/07/$ - see front matter
doi:10.1016/j.pmr.2007.03.004

Adipose tissue is a specialized connective tissue that is comprised of lipid-filled cells (adipocytes) contained within a collagen framework. The adipocyte is 90% triglycerides, with small amounts of diglycerides, monoglycerides, cholesterol, phospholipids, free fatty acids, protein, and water. Its primary function is as a reservoir for stored energy, but it also serves as a mechanical cushion and insulator for heat conservation. Adipose tissue is the least heavy of the stored energy substrates within the human body, with a molecular density of 0.901 g/mL, although with 9 kcal/g of tissue, it has a much higher energy density than either carbohydrate (4 kcal/g) or protein (4 kcal/g). Storing energy as fat in the human body therefore provides much better mobility because of its high energy and low molecular density [2].

Fat storage (lipogenesis) occurs from the processing of primary foodstuffs during parasympathetic-mediated postprandial conditions. Carbohydrates, proteins, and fats are processed in the digestive tract and immediately used for reparative and metabolic functions or are stored as future fuel sources. Only small amounts of carbohydrates are stored as glycogen in muscle (150 g) and liver (90 g), and even smaller amounts are used for immediate metabolism and repair. Excess carbohydrates are converted to fat and stored efficiently as adipose tissue. Similarly, ingested protein is digested into amino acids, and those that are not immediately incorporated into structural proteins, hormones, or enzymes are converted into adipose tissue, with the excess nitrogen excreted in the urine and feces. Dietary fat and cholesterol is readily digested and packaged into water-soluble chylomicrons, which can be transported to the liver and adipocytes for processing and storage. Regardless of foodstuff composition, a diet high in caloric density will ultimately result in adipose accumulation when energy needs are sufficiently met. As the energy system is stressed in times of relative famine, carbohydrates and proteins are actually catabolized sooner and at higher rates than adipose tissue. Subsequently, attempts to diet for rapid weight loss often result in early loss of water, protein, and carbohydrates with relatively small amounts of adipose reduction. Because the protein stores used come primarily from skeletal muscle, resting metabolism is subsequently reduced after rapid weight loss, resulting in a lower rate of energy expenditure at rest and during exercise that ultimately favors accumulation of more energy storage (ie, adipose tissue).

As rates of obesity increased within the United States, the World Health Organization (WHO) began to take note and, in the mid-1990s, began to look for an easier method to identify persons at risk than the labor-intensive body composition assessment tools used by early researchers. Impressive data had been collected in the United States by the National Health and Nutrition Examination Surveys (NHANES I-III) in three different cycles, using height and weight to correlate obesity with morbidity and mortality. In 1998, the WHO introduced the use of body mass index (BMI) as a screening tool to stratify persons for risk of obesity-related disorders. BMI is determined by dividing weight (kg) by height (m) squared, and has been used by American insurance companies for decades to predict risk for morbidity and mortality. According to the WHO definitions, BMI less than 18 kg/m^2 is considered underweight, 18 to 24.9 kg/m^2 is normal weight, 25 to 29.9 kg/m^2 is overweight, and greater than 30 kg/m^2 is obese. In recent years, additional classifications for moderate (30–34.9 kg/m^2), severe (35–39.9 kg/m^2), and very severe (>40 kg/m^2) obesity have also been added, reflecting exponentially increased risk for hypertension, hyperlipidemia, heart disease, and diabetes. BMI is easily calculated in most populations with minimal time, expense, and effort, and therefore provides a simple and efficient way to collect epidemiologic data and stratify risk. Unfortunately, BMI lacks the sensitivity to differentiate body fat from fat-free lean mass (FFM). Therefore, a large, muscular athlete who has only 4%BF but a BMI of 31 kg/m^2 would be inappropriately classified as obese according to the WHO definition. Conversely, a person who has tetraplegia might have normal weight relative to height, but have 38%BF despite a BMI of 25 kg/m^2. This relationship will be discussed in more detail later.

Genetics or environment

Obesity is the result of a complex interaction between genetic predisposition and environmental factors that can be altered to favor the accumulation of adipose tissue. Familial tendencies toward obesity have been shown in both animal and human models. Recent investigations have shown an association or link to phenotypic obesity in more than 600 genes, markers, or regions on all potential loci except the Y human chromosome [3]. The "thrifty gene theory" suggests this is an evolutionary adaptation to favor energy storage for times of famine [4,5], although the way in which fat is distributed varies among individuals and imparts different risk. Android (apple-shape) obesity is associated with greater cardiovascular risk and seems to be caused by a genetic predisposition to accumulate visceral (central) adipose tissue, whereas persons who have a genetic predisposition for gynoid (pear-shape) obesity more rapidly accumulate fat stores in the hips and thighs, with less risk for cardiovascular consequences [6]. An estimated heritability for obesity of between 50% to 90% falls well short of explaining the rapid increase in societal obesity over the past 20 years, suggesting that phenotypic expression of specific genomes can be drastically influenced by environmental factors. Specific factors contributing to this trend include diminished physical activity, increasingly frequent sedentary choices for leisure activity, and easy access to highly palatable, high-caloric, low-nutrient density foods in America's industrialized society [7].

Adipose tissue is especially likely to accumulate in four periods of life: infancy, childhood, adolescence, and pregnancy. Adipocytes are size-dependent. As the adipocyte hypertrophies beyond a certain size, it divides into two separate cells, which can again hypertrophy and divide during periods of positive energy balance. Although adipocytes can atrophy during periods of famine and negative energy balance, the hyperplasia is irreversible and seems to increase the body's "set point" to a higher level of adiposity; rapid adipocyte accumulation therefore increases one's risk for lifelong obesity. During fetal development and infancy, adipose accumulation is limited by the mother's nutrient availability, whereas childhood adipose accumulation additionally increases in response to human growth hormone and insulin-like growth factors. Adolescent lipogenesis increases directly with sex steroid concentrations and nutrient availability, whereas further changes in hormonal fluctuations mediate adipose accumulation during maternal pregnancy. Although these periods of rapid fat accumulation seem integral to lifelong obesity, experts have also recognized that chronic periods of positive energy balance beyond these critical periods can also contribute to adiposity and adipose hyperplasia.

The concept of energy balance reflects an ever-dynamic relationship between relative rates of change for energy intake and energy expenditure. When discussing these parameters, the term *Calorie* is typically used, although when written with a capital C it actually represents kilocalories. A single Calorie is the amount of energy required to increase the temperature of 1 kg water by 1°C at 1 atmosphere pressure. Energy intake reflects the caloric gain through ingestion of foodstuffs, whereas energy expenditure reflects calories used to sustain life, perform movement, and digest food.

Energy intake is provided through the ingestion of foodstuffs of varying caloric densities. Fats contain roughly 9 kcal/g, carbohydrates and proteins contain approximately 4 kcal/g and alcohol contains approximately 7 kcal/g. The perceived need for energy is mediated through the lateral (appetite center) and ventromedial (satiety center) nuclei of the hypothalamus. These centers summate influences from various circulating substrates, hormones, neuropeptides, and neurotransmitter signals. Insulin, leptin, and several gastrointestinal substances, including cholecystokinin (CCK), glucagon-like peptide-1 (GLP-1), apolipoprotein A-IV (Apo-A-IV), insulin, and glucose are known to suppress appetite, whereas cortisol and ghrelin increase in the preprandial state and stimulate appetite and food intake [1]. However, nonphysiologic external factors, such as emotional state, food characteristics, lifestyle behaviors, and environmental cues, can override the summation of appetite and satiety signals, compromising the delicate balance of metabolic homeostasis [8]. For example, these external factors can and often do increase the release of orexigenic (appetite-stimulating) neuropeptides from the hypothalamus, even during periods of positive energy balance, resulting in the additional accumulation of adipose tissue despite physiologic cues of satiation.

In periods of metabolic homeostasis (ie, energy balance), energy expenditure will equally offset energy intake. Energy expenditure is the sum of basal metabolic rate (BMR), the thermic effect of food digestion (TEF), and the thermic effect of physical activity (TEA). Of the three, BMR contributes the most to total daily energy expenditure (TDEE), representing approximately

60% to 70% of the total. BMR represents the minimal energy expenditure required to sustain life, and equations developed around the beginning of the 20th century remain in use, although modified in recent decades to reflect a larger anthropometric body type [9]. Still more recent investigations have indicated those modified equations actually overestimate basal energy expenditure in most adults, particularly those who have increasingly sedentary lifestyles [10]. FFM, comprised of muscle, bone, and organs, contributes the greatest energy expenditure of the basal metabolic rate, and of the FFM components, skeletal muscle contributes up to 85% of the variance [11,12]. Therefore, increases or decreases in skeletal muscle mass significantly impact not only caloric expenditure during activity but also total energy expenditure at rest. The TEF is the least variable of the components of TDEE, because digestion, absorption, and sympathetic nervous system activation after consumption of foodstuffs remains constant with normal physiology and does not depend on body weight or composition. TEF represent approximately 8% of TDEE in most individuals [13]. Intermediate and most variable among the components of TDEE is the thermic effect of activity. Not only does it depend on total body mass and skeletal muscle mass, it varies significantly with the mode, intensity, duration, and frequency of activities performed.

Regardless of genetic influences, a person's energy balance is profoundly impacted by SCI. Injury to the somatic nervous system results in immediate and sustained loss of neurotrophic influences to skeletal muscles below the level of SCI, whereas sympathetic blunting in injuries above T6 further impairs energy metabolism. Paralyzed muscle atrophies rapidly (obligatory sarcopenia) after acute SCI, drastically reducing BMR and TEA directly with the level of injury, and therefore higher levels of SCI result in greater reductions in BMR and TEA. TEA is further reduced in traumatic SCI because of activity, range of motion (ROM), and weight-bearing restrictions associated with surgical repair and bony healing. Subsequently, predicted energy expenditure equations used to determine caloric and nitrogen needs overestimate actual needs by an average of approximately 25% in persons who have new SCI. These reductions are sustained after the acute phase of SCI [14–20], because of reduced FFM, sympathetic blunting, cardiopulmonary dysfunction, reductions in work capacity, diminished anabolic hormones, and reduced ability to use the large muscle mass of the lower extremities. If equivalent reductions in energy intake are not provided, people who have SCI will rapidly accumulate adipose tissue beyond that expected of non-SCI individuals in similar circumstances. Modifying components of energy intake and energy expenditure to promote metabolic homeostasis are discussed in more detail later.

Pathophysiology of adipose tissue

Once considered benign, adipose tissue has recently been shown to mediate severe metabolic consequences when accumulated in excess and has been implicated as the causative agent for cardiovascular inflammation, hyperlipidemia, insulin resistance, hypertension, and thromboemboli [21].

Adipose tissue, particularly that in visceral regions, has been shown to secrete large amounts of proinflammatory proteins called cytokines, including interleukin-6 (IL-6) and tumor-necrosis factor-α (TNF-α) [22]. IL-6 is a potent proinflammatory cytokine released from visceral and subcutaneous adipocytes that independently causes low-grade vascular inflammation, stimulates the release of cortisol from the adrenal cortex, and stimulates hepatic production of C-reactive protein (CRP), an acute-phase reactant that is also associated with vascular inflammation. TNF-α is also a proinflammatory protein released in large quantities from adipocytes that independently causes low-grade vascular inflammation and similarly facilitates the synthesis of acute-phase reactants, CRP, and fibrinogen [23,24]. The amplified effect of these adipocyte-derived cytokines leads directly and indirectly to vascular endothelial cell injury and apoptosis [25].

Few studies have investigated the proinflammatory state of the vascular tree in SCI [26,27]. Lee and colleagues [27] recently reported elevated CRP levels in the high-risk range for a convenience sample of veterans with SCI, 22.6% of which were classified with metabolic syndrome using conservative standards. Insulin resistance was reported in 22% of the sample; however, body composition was not reported. Manns and colleagues [26] also reported CRP levels in the high-risk range for 22 individuals who had paraplegia and a mean %BF of 26.7. IL-6 and TNF- have not yet been reported in the SCI population.

As adipose tissue accumulates, lipolysis that typically occurs in the fasted state produces nonesterified fatty acids (NEFA) at an accelerated rate, even with rising insulin levels. Circulating NEFA are deposited in the liver and skeletal muscle at increasing rates, contributing to insulin resistance by inhibiting the phosphorylation of insulin receptor substrates (IRS-1 and IRS-2) and subsequently the phosphatidylinositol 3-kinase (PI-3 kinase) cascade necessary for activation of the GLUT1 and GLUT4 receptors that allow them to translocate to the cell membrane and facilitate passage of glucose into the cell [28]. As NEFA and associated triglycerides accumulate within the liver, hepatic production of very–low-density (VLDL) and low-density (LDL) lipoproteins increases, as does that of apolipoprotein B, the major protein of LDL-cholesterol (LDL-c) [29,30]. Simultaneously, net apolipoprotein A production is slowed, resulting in reductions of high-density lipoprotein (HDL), the primary scavenger of peripheral lipids [29]. Whole-body lipid profiles reflect the local hepatic changes in lipid metabolism with elevated triglycerides, very–low-density lipoprotein cholesterol (VLDL-c), LDL and LDL-c in the face of diminishing high-density lipoprotein cholesterol (HDL-c), creating an atherogenic environment throughout the vascular tree [31]. These relationships seem clearly related to adiposity in SCI, with low HDL-c, elevated triglycerides, and elevated LDL-c reported in numerous investigations [26,27,32–36].

Circulating NEFA and triglycerides secreted from excess adipose tissue contribute to insulin resistance. Specifically, fatty acid metabolites (ceramide and diacylglycerol) within muscle and liver cells impair the PI 3-kinase cascade, ultimately reducing glucose transport into the cells because of impaired glucose transporter types 1 and 4 (GLUT1 and GLUT4) receptor translocation to the cell membranes [28,37]. In addition, the inflammatory cytokines IL-6 and TNF-α inhibit the proximal portion of the insulin signaling cascade, further contributing to insulin resistance [38]. Subsequently, insulin release from pancreatic β cells is chronically increased, resulting in simultaneous hyperinsulinemia and hyperglycemia, until the β cells ultimately fail in response to chronic hyperstimulation. Insulin resistance in SCI has been reported in several manuscripts, most of which have also shown a strong relationship with %BF [20,26,27,34,39,40].

Central obesity causes hypertension through several mechanisms. Chronic exposure to adipose-derived proinflammatory cytokines can damage the arterial endothelium, resulting in arterial stiffness and dysfunction. Visceral fat also secretes the hormone leptin, which directly increases sympathetic nervous system activity, increasing vasoconstriction and subsequently mean arterial pressure [41,42]. Adipocyte secretion of TNF-α increases hepatic synthesis of angiotensinogen, a potent vasoconstrictive agent [43]. Recent evidence shows that angiotensinogen is also released directly from adipocytes, further amplifying the renin–angiotensin–aldosterone system (RAAS) and contributing to systemic hypertension [43]. Specifically, these agents stimulate aldosterone production from the adrenal cortex with subsequent renal sodium reabsorption and volume expansion [44]. Visceral obesity can also cause direct mechanical compression of the kidneys, causing elevated intrarenal pressures and sodium retention [42]. Along with the vasoconstrictive properties of angiotensinogen, systemic hypertension results. In persons who have SCI, these effects may be ameliorated with sympathetic blunting, which subsequently diminishes vascular tone and results in neurogenic hypotension. Despite SCI neuropathophysiology, hypertension has recently been reported in 22% of a large veteran cohort with SCI; 68% of the cohort had a BMI greater than 23 kg/m^2, suggesting a relationship between hypertension and obesity [45].

To complete the atherogenic picture painted by obesity, adipocytes have recently been associated with two powerful prothrombotic agents that increase the risk for blood clotting in the vascular tree. Plasminogen activator inhibitor (PAI-1) is directly secreted from adipocytes and is a potent inhibitor of fibrinolysis; PAI-1 concentration is increased in direct proportion to total adipose mass [46–48]. Thrombin-activatable fibrinolysis inhibitor (TAFI) has also been directly associated with adipose mass, although it is secreted primarily from the liver in response to elevated circulating lipids [47,48]. Both agents have been shown to impair fibrinolysis and increase risk for thromboemboli. Neither substance has been reported in the SCI literature.

Collectively, the constellation of obesity, vascular inflammation, dyslipidemia, insulin resistance, and hypertension has been referred to as a "metabolic syndrome," although the relative impact of each component on overall health has been debated among physicians and scientists. In 1998, the WHO definition of the metabolic syndrome focused on the central role of diabetes mellitus plus at least two of the following: obesity (BMI or waist-to-hip ratios), dyslipidemia (TG $\geq$150 mg/dL and/or HDL-c $<$35 mg/dL in men or $<$39 mg/dL in women), hypertension (blood pressure $\geq$140/90 mm Hg), and microalbuminuria [49]. The third panel of the National Cholesterol Education Project (ATP III) definition of the metabolic syndrome placed equal emphasis on any three of the following: obesity (waist circumference $\geq$102 cm in men, or $\geq$88 cm in women), dyslipidemia (TG $\geq$150 mg/dL and/or HDL-c $<$40 mg/dL in men or $<$50 mg/dL in women), hypertension (BP $\geq$130/85 mm Hg), and fasting glucose greater than 110 mg/dL [50]. Most recently, the International Diabetes Federation (IDF) definition of metabolic syndrome has emphasized the role of central obesity (waist circumference $\geq$94 cm in men or $\geq$80 cm in women) plus any two of the following: dyslipidemia (TG $\geq$150 mg/dL or on treatment; HDL-c $<$40 mg/dL for men or $<$50 mg/dL for women or on HDL-c treatment), hypertension ($\geq$130 mm Hg systolic or $\geq$85 mm Hg diastolic, or on treatment for hypertension), and fasting glucose of 100 mg/dL or higher [51]. Obesity is now recognized as the primary mediator of the metabolic consequences of this syndrome.

In addition to its metabolic consequences, obesity has been correlated with several other pathological states, as shown in Box 1. Even without SCI, persons who have obesity are at high risk for developing osteoarthritis. The risk for osteoarthritis at hips, knees, and ankles is greater in persons with incomplete SCI who are able to ambulate with or without assistive devices because of abnormal joint forces associated with spasticity, reduced proprioception, and neurogenic gait dynamics. For persons with SCI who rely on the upper extremities for mobility and transfers, upper extremity overuse is a significant issue that is further exacerbated by obesity [52]. The shoulder is particularly at risk in persons with SCI who rely on their upper extremities for wheelchair propulsion and transfers in and out of their chairs; numerous studies have shown a high incidence of osteoarthritis and rotator cuff dysfunction in this vulnerable population [53–62]. The incidence of carpal tunnel syndrome (CTS) is increased in persons who are obese [63–65] and in persons who have SCI [62,66,67]; that the symptoms of CTS would be worse under conditions of both obesity and SCI with mobility at stake is a reasonable assumption. Recent studies show that ulnar neuropathies are also a significant risk for wheelchair users [68,69]. As upper-extremity pain and dysfunction occurs, activity patterns typically decrease, resulting in further reductions in energy expenditure and subsequent weight gain [52]. Several morbidities listed in Box 1 have not been solidly linked to obesity in persons who have SCI, although the author believes this is because of lack of investigation rather than lack of relation.

Box 1. Dangers associated with obesity

Angina pectoris
Breast cancer
Carpal tunnel syndrome
Cerebrovascular accidents
Cholecystitis/cholelithiasis
Colon cancer
Congestive heart failure
Coronary artery disease
Depression
Diabetes mellitus/glucose intolerance
Dyslipidemia
Gout
Hyperinsulinemia/insulin resistance
Nephrolithiasis
Obstructive sleep apnea
Osteoarthritis
Peripheral vascular disease
Pressure ulcers
Reproductive dysfunction
Social isolation

Prevalence of obesity in spinal cord injury

The author believes that obesity is present in more than two thirds of persons who have SCI, although limited data are available supporting that assumption, largely because of inappropriate characterization of obesity in the SCI population. When the WHO redefined obesity according to BMI in 1998, significant sensitivity for the true definition of obesity [70] (%BF >22 in men and %BF >35 in women) was compromised, resulting in gross underestimation of obesity in certain populations, including those who had SCI [2]. Additionally, standard body composition assessment techniques are based on non-SCI cadaveric dissections performed more than 50 years ago and have not been validated in the SCI population [71]. Limitations for each of the current techniques used for body composition assessment in SCI were reported previously [71].

In brief, underwater (hydrostatic) weighing assumptions that the components of FFM (water, protein, and mineral) are proportionally constant and do not differ from the "reference" man are violated in SCI, and residual lung volumes are significantly greater and must be accurately measured when determining body density. Body density using air displacement plethysmography was validated against hydrostatic weighing, and similarly violates those assumptions. Additionally, the author has reported the inability to register accurate thoracic gas volumes for persons who have SCI above T6, which further limits application of this technique in SCI [72]. Hydrometry also relies on assumptions from the hydrostatic weighing model, and further assumes no abnormal fluid shifts (eg, lower-extremity edema, venous pooling) are present; these assumptions are violated in the SCI population. Dual-energy x-ray absorptiometry (DXA) similarly relies on assumptions made for hydrostatic weighing, assumes constant hydration, and further assumes that fat content in unmeasured pixels (ie, those underlying and overlying bone) is the same as that in measured pixels. The latter assumption is especially problematic in persons who have SCI, because the ratios between lower-extremity tissue girth and bone diameter are significantly reduced from muscle atrophy, whereas the unchanged tissue girth–to–bone diameter ratios in the upper extremities and trunk underrepresent bone-free pixels because of the large areas of bone in these regions. More than 60% of the 21,000 pixels in a typical whole-body DXA scan are estimated to contain bone, and are therefore excluded from the calculation of values for soft tissues in persons who have SCI; adipose tissue overlying and underlying bone is not included, and is subsequently underestimated [71]. Bioelectrical impedance analyses (BIA) has also been used to estimate body composition in persons who have SCI, but similarly relies on assumptions from hydrostatic weighing by which it was derived. Like hydrometry and DXA, BIA for body composition assessment assumes constant fluid compartments in persons who have SCI; violation of these assumptions similarly invalidates its use in the SCI population. Finally, anthropometry (limb widths, lengths, girths, circumferences and skinfold thicknesses) has been used to estimate body composition using hydrostatic weighing as a reference. Anthropometric equations are population-specific and no equations specific to persons who have SCI have been validated. To accurately assess body composition in these individuals, four-compartment modeling is required, which separately determines body density, total body water, bone mineral content, and subsequently derived fat. Recommendations for reporting SCI body composition and obesity in future clinical trials have been provided previously [71].

Only one study has reported SCI body composition by four-compartment modeling in the literature, showing that 10 of 13 persons (77%) who had paraplegia had %BF in the obese range, even though mean BMI was less than 25 kg/m^2 [72]. Table 1 shows recent SCI studies that have reported %BF and BMI. Even those studies showing mean BMI in the low 20s reported mean %BF in the obese range [15,19,20,72–79]. One study has recently shown that 133 men who had SCI were on average 13% fatter (as determined with DXA) than age-, height-, and ethnicity-matched non-SCI controls [20]. These data indicate that for persons who have SCI and BMI greater than 25 kg/m^2, obesity is clearly present; even athletic populations with SCI and BMI of 22 kg/m^2 are obese according to hydrostatic weighing, which is known to underestimate %BF in this population [73,75].

Table 1
Demographics, body mass index, and percent body fat in recent spinal cord injury trials

Authors	N	Age (y)	Body mass index (kg/m^2)	% Fat	Spinal chord injury
Buchholz et al [15]	28	34.2	24.3	30.8	Para
Bulbulian et al [73]	22	27.5	22.3	22.4	Para
Clasey and Gater [72]	13	37	24.8	27	Para
Desport et al [74]	20	45.4	26.9	32.8	Para
George et al [75]	15	30.8	22.3	25.5	Para/tetra
Jones et al [76]	20	16–52	23.1	27.5	Para
	7	16–52	26.7	35	Tetra
Maggioni et al [77]	12	33.8	25.7	31.1	Para
Modlesky et al [78]	8	35	24.6	33.8	Para
Monroe et al [79]	10	31.9	21.7	23	Para
Spungen et al [19]	8	40	22.3	33.5	Para
Spungen et al [20]	67	40	25.4	36.3	Para
	66	37	25.8	34.2	Tetra

Abbreviations: Para, paraplegic; tetra, tetraplegic.

The true prevalence of obesity in SCI remains questionable, but the reader is asked to consider the following. In a sample of 7959 veterans who had SCI managed in Veterans Affairs (VA) hospitals in 2001, 53% were reported to have BMI greater than 25 kg/m^2, whereas 68% had BMI greater than 23 kg/m^2 [45]. A smaller sample reported from a single mid-western VA hospital similarly showed that 255 (65.8%) of 387 veterans who had SCI had BMI greater than 25 kg/m^2; an additional 27.9% were reported to have BMI in the normal range (20–25 kg/m^2). The studies reported previously suggest that at least half of the individuals who have SCI and normal BMIs would also fall into the obese range if %BF were accurately assessed. Unfortunately, other large epidemiologic databases specific to SCI outside the VA system have not collected heights and weights, and therefore even gross measures of obesity using BMI cannot be determined. Nonetheless, when considering the data presented in Table 1 with those of the two large studies, the best data currently available suggest that two of every three persons who have SCI are likely obese and appear at risk for the metabolic consequences of obesity.

Management of obesity in spinal cord injury

Treatment of obesity in SCI remains largely empiric, because few studies have actually investigated obesity management in this vulnerable population [80]. Simplistically, reductions in energy intake, increases in metabolic rate, and increased energy expenditure would result in a negative energy balance, with subsequent reductions in adipose tissue. The difficulty lies in knowing what the total daily energy expenditure (TDEE) is for each individual. As indicated previously, TDEE in persons who have SCI is reduced by 12% to 54%, depending on level of injury, FFM, and activity level

[14–16,79,81]. Cox and colleagues [16] provided estimates of energy intake parameters for persons who have paraplegia (27.9 kcal/kg/d) and tetraplegia (22.7 kcal/kg/d) based on a small sample, but did not control for spasticity, wounds, hormones, autonomic dysreflexia, or other factors that could impact the TDEE. This study has not been replicated. Current recommendations are to use individualized indirect calorimetry to determine energy needs for persons who have SCI until energy expenditure prediction equations specific to SCI have been developed and validated [82]. When the TDEE is known, the options can be assessed for changing energy intake through diet and energy expenditure through exercise to determine what is most reasonable for the individual.

Dietary management of obesity in SCI is challenging, because the TDEE is much reduced [82]. As recommended previously, physicians must be careful not to overfeed in the acute setting, recognizing that obligatory nitrogen loss associated with paralysis cannot be diminished through excess calorie administration with or without high protein [17,18]. Failure to recognize this early in SCI will likely lead to a significant shift in body composition with excess adipose tissue replacing lost muscle because of continued overfeeding. The recent Dietary Guidelines of America (DGA) have made general recommendations for adults who are at normal or overweight, and include both dietary guidelines and activity recommendations [83]. Greater emphasis is placed on the ingestion of nutrient dense foods that limit saturated and trans fats, cholesterol, added sugars, salt, and alcohol. Furthermore, foods with a high glycemic index, such as juice, soda, baked goods, candy, sweetened cereals, canned fruits with syrup, and dried fruits, should be avoided because they rapidly increase insulin secretion and subsequently facilitate lipogenesis and hyperinsulinemia. Low-fat diets (approximately 28% of total calories) with complex rather than simple carbohydrates have been shown to promote modest, sustainable weight loss [84]. Rapid weight-loss diets are discouraged, because they promote additional muscle loss and dehydration, resulting in further reductions of basal metabolism that typically preclude future attempts at weight maintenance and energy balance [85]. Successful diets (those that facilitate future weight maintenance) usually promote reductions of caloric intake sufficient to allow negative energy balance of 100 to 200 kcal/d, with weight loss of approximately 1 to 2 lb/wk. Restaurant eating is generally discouraged, but if individuals must dine out regularly, they should (1) select restaurants with low-fat and healthy food options, (2) request less fat in food preparation, dressing on the side, and no butter, (3) avoid all-you-can-eat buffets, (4) pre-plan what they will order before arriving, (5) avoid large portions, split portions with a companion or ask the server to place half in a "doggie" bag before starting, and leave food on their plates, and (6) ask the server to remove tempting foods from the table when enough has been consumed [86]. Limiting alcoholic beverages can also reduce empty calories (ie, those with no nutrient value).

Exercise is often recommended for weight loss, but too often is not prescribed with sufficient detail to be useful to the participant. The DGA recently suggested that 60 min/d of moderate to vigorous physical activity above normal activities is required to prevent continuous weight gain, and that 90 min/d of moderate to vigorous activity seems necessary to prevent weight gain in persons who were previously overweight or obese. To lose weight, the DGA recommend 90 minutes of moderate to vigorous activity above normal activities most days of the week. In practical terms, moderate to vigorous exercise has been defined as working with sufficient intensity to warrant speaking in three- to five-word sentences [87]. If one cannot get at least three words out between breaths during exercise, the intensity is too high. If one can speak more than five words between breaths, the intensity is too low. Benefits from exercise include weight loss, increased FFM (including muscle and bone), reduced fat mass, improved strength, improved endurance, improved cardiovascular fitness, and improvements in psychosocial factors. The extent to which each of these benefits is achieved depends on the mode, frequency, intensity, and duration applied.

Exercise prescription for persons who have SCI should be directed toward specific client goals, and appropriate risk-factor analysis should be completed before they participate in a moderate to vigorous exercise program [87]. Contraindications and limitations to exercise in SCI include blunted sympathetic responses caused by autonomic dysfunction, neurogenic hypotension, circulatory hypokinesis, adaptive myocardial atrophy with reduced cardiac output, impaired cardiac chronotropic/inotropic capacity, reduced tidal volumes, bronchiolar constriction, impaired ventilatory capacity, upper-extremity overuse syndrome, impaired upper- and lower-extremity proprioception, spasticity, osteopenia/osteoporosis, neurogenic skin, neurogenic bowel, neurogenic bladder, impaired thermoregulation, and autonomic dysreflexia [87–89]. If goals include strengthening, weight loss, or body composition improvement, the exercise prescription could incorporate resistance exercise and aerobic conditioning [89]. Too often, resistance training for FFM gain in SCI is overlooked, and it has significant implications for increasing TDEE because muscle is metabolically active tissue [11,12]. Increasing FFM might have a greater overall impact on TDEE than aerobic exercise, because it would increase BMR 24 h/d, whereas the energy expenditure of aerobic exercise is mostly restricted to the exercise bout itself and the immediate postexercise period.

Most exercise studies involving persons who have SCI have focused on outcome variables for cardiopulmonary fitness, strength, endurance, and some combination of risk factors, including dyslipidemia and glucose tolerance, without emphasizing adipose reduction [87,89]. Few studies have even attempted to measure changes in %BF in response to exercise, and only modest improvements have been reported for those that have used lower-extremity functional electrical stimulation [90,91]. The author is aware of no reported upper-extremity strength or conditioning studies in SCI that have reported improvements in %BF. This may be caused by the intensive labor required for appropriate body composition assessment and the lack of emphasis on exercise for adipose reduction in the SCI population.

The combination of diet and exercise is the most logical approach to reduce obesity in SCI. Diet alone may result in diminished TDEE because of reductions in FFM, whereas exercise alone may not increase TDEE sufficiently to offset caloric intake. In most non-SCI populations, the combination of diet and exercise has almost always resulted in greater loss of body fat while sustaining or improving FFM, with superior results for long-term weight maintenance. Similar results are expected for persons who have SCI, although little information is currently available. Chen and colleagues [80] provided a 12-week behavioral intervention program to 16 individuals who had SCI and reported a small but significant difference in BMI, fat mass, and waist circumference, with increased HDL-c that persisted 12 weeks after completion. The program consisted primarily of education and was not strictly controlled in diet or exercise interventions, although it included both.

Pharmacologic intervention for obesity in SCI has not been reported in the literature. Current formulations, such as sibutramine and orlistat, that have been approved for obesity management in the non-SCI population have not been tested in persons who have SCI, and have potentially harmful side-effects in this special population. Sibutramine blocks norepinephrine and serotonin reuptake and may overstimulate the central nervous system because of up-regulation of postsynaptic catecholamine receptors in SCI [92]. Orlistat inhibits pancreatic lipase and blocks intestinal lipid absorption, which could lead to uncontrolled steatorrhea, silent cramping, and autonomic dysreflexia in persons who have neurogenic bowel [93]. Although several other medications, including phentermine, diethylpropion, fluoxetine, sertraline, bupropion, topiramate, and zonisamide, have been evaluated for obesity management, data are currently insufficient to recommend their use, particularly because no data have assessed their use in SCI [93–95]. Amphetamines and their derivatives are not appropriate for weight loss in SCI.

Finally, interventional trials for surgical options such as gastric stapling, fat reduction, and liposuction have not been reported in the population with SCI, although guidelines are available for individuals who do not have SCI [94]. These procedures are associated with significant risk and cannot be recommended for use in individuals who have SCI until safety and efficacy have been established.

Summary

Obesity is at epidemic proportions in the population with SCI and is likely the mediator of the metabolic syndrome in this special population. It has been poorly appreciated in SCI largely because of the lack of sensitivity BMI conveys for obesity risk in SCI. Recent studies in non-SCI populations have shown the causal relationship between adipose tissue accumulation and vascular inflammation, dyslipidemia, insulin resistance/glucose intolerance, hypertension, and thromboemboli. Similar findings have been seen in persons who have SCI, although the causative link with adipose tissue has not been previously reported. Management options remain largely empiric and behavioral, and recommendations for appropriate dietary intervention and exercise counseling remain the mainstay of treatment, despite the lack of evidence for these interventions in SCI.

References

[1] Bray GA, Fisler J, York DA. Neuroendocrine control of the development of obesity—understanding gained from studies of experimental animal-models. Front Neuroendocrinol 1990;11(2):128–81.

[2] Gater D. Pathophysiology of obesity after spinal cord injury. Top Spinal Cord Inj Rehabil 2007;12(4):20–34.

[3] Perusse L, Rankinen T, Zuberi A, et al. The human obesity gene map: the 2004 update. Obes Res 2005;13(3):381–490.

[4] Clement K, Ferre P. Genetics and the pathophysiology of obesity. Pediatr Res 2003;53(5): 721–5.

[5] Cummings DE, Schwartz MW. Genetics and pathophysiology of human obesity. Annu Rev Med 2003;54:453–71.

[6] Terry RB, Stefanick ML, Haskell WL, et al. Contributions of regional adipose-tissue depots to plasma-lipoprotein concentrations in overweight men and women—possible protective effects of thigh fat. Metab Clin Exp 1991;40(7):733–40.

[7] Hill JO, Peters JC. Environmental contributions to the obesity epidemic. Science 1998; 280(5368):1371–4.

[8] Schwartz MW, Woods SC, Porte D, et al. Central nervous system control of food intake. Nature 2000;404(6778):661–71.

[9] Schofield W. Predicting basal metablic rate, new standards and review of previous work. Hum Nutr Clin Nutr 1985;39(Suppl):5–41.

[10] Alfonzo-Gonzalez G, Doucet E, Almeras N, et al. Estimation of daily energy needs with the FAO/WHO/UNU 1985 procedures in adults: comparison to whole-body indirect calorimetry measurements. Eur J Clin Nutr 2004;58(8):1125–31.

[11] Illner K, Brinkmann G, Heller M, et al. Metabolically active components of fat free mass and resting energy expenditure in nonobese adults. Am J Physiol Endocrinol Metab 2000;278(2): E308–15.

[12] Sparti A, DeLany JP, de la Bretonne JA, et al. Relationship between resting metabolic rate and the composition of the fat-free mass. Metabolism 1997;46(10):1225–30.

[13] Segal KR, Presta E, Gutin B. Thermic effect of food during graded-exercise in normal weight and obese men. Am J Clin Nutr 1984;40(5):995–1000.

[14] Bauman WA, Spungen AM, Wang J, et al. The relationship between energy expenditure and lean tissue in monozygotic twins discordant for spinal cord injury. J Rehabil Res Dev 2004; 41(1):1–8.

[15] Buchholz AC, McGillivray CF, Pencharz PB. Differences in resting metabolic rate between paraplegic and able-bodied subjects are explained by differences in body composition. Am J Clin Nutr 2003;77(2):371–8.

[16] Cox SAR, Weiss SM, Posuniak EA, et al. Energy-expenditure after spinal-cord injury—an evaluation of stable rehabilitating patients. J Trauma 1985;25(5):419–23.

[17] Rodriguez DJ, Clevenger FW, Osler TM, et al. Obligatory negative nitrogen-balance following spinal-cord injury. JPEN J Parenter Enteral Nutr 1991;15(3):319–22.

[18] Rodriguez DJ, Benzel EC, Clevenger FW. The metabolic response to spinal cord injury. Spinal Cord 1997;35(9):599–604.

[19] Spungen AM, Wang J, Pierson RN, et al. Soft tissue body composition differences in monozygotic twins discordant for spinal cord injury. J Appl Physiol 2000;88(4):1310–5.
[20] Spungen AM, Adkins RH, Stewart CA, et al. Factors influencing body composition in persons with spinal cord injury: a cross-sectional study. J Appl Physiol 2003;95(6):2398–407.
[21] Grundy SM. Obesity, metabolic syndrome, and cardiovascular disease. J Clin Endocrinol Metab 2004;89(6):2595–600.
[22] Matsuzawa Y. White adipose tissue and cardiovascular disease. Best Pract Research Clin Endocrinol Metab 2005;19(4):637–47.
[23] Kern PA, Saghizadeh M, Ong JM, et al. The expression of tumor-necrosis-factor in human adipose-tissue—regulation by obesity, weight-loss, and relationship to lipoprotein-lipase. J Clin Invest 1995;95(5):2111–9.
[24] Kern PA, Ranganathan S, Li CL, et al. Adipose tissue tumor necrosis factor and interleukin-6 expression in human obesity and insulin resistance. Am J Physiol Endocrinol Metab 2001; 280(5):E745–51.
[25] Blake GJ, Ridker PM. Novel clinical markers of vascular wall inflammation. Circ Res 2001; 89(9):763–71.
[26] Manns PJ, McCubbin JA, Williams DP. Fitness, inflammation, and the metabolic syndrome in men with paraplegia. Arch Phys Med Rehabil 2005;86(6):1176–81.
[27] Lee MY, Myers J, Hayes A, et al. C-reactive protein, metabolic syndrome, and insulin resistance in individuals with spinal cord injury. J Spinal Cord Med 2005;28(1):20–5.
[28] Shulman GI. Cellular mechanisms of insulin resistance. J Clin Invest 2000;106(2):171–6.
[29] Kolovou GD, Anagnostopoulou KK, Cokkinos DV. Pathophysiology of dyslipidaemia in the metabolic syndrome. Postgrad Med J 2005;81(956):358–66.
[30] Kwiterovich PO Jr, Coresh J, Bachorik PS. Prevalence of hyperapobetalipoproteinemia and other lipoprotein phenotypes in men (aged < or = 50 years) and women(< or = 60 years) with coronary artery disease. Am J Cardiol 1993;71(8):631–9.
[31] Verges B. New insight into the pathophysiology of lipid abnormalities in type 2 diabetes. Diabetes Metab 2005;31(5):429–39.
[32] Bauman WA, Adkins RH, Spungen AM, et al. Is immobilization associated with an abnormal lipoprotein profile? Observations from a diverse cohort. Spinal Cord 1999;37(7):485–93.
[33] Dallmeijer AJ, Hopman MT, Van der Woude LH. Lipid, lipoprotein, and apolipoprotein profiles in active and sedentary men with tetraplegia. Arch Phys Med Rehabil 1997; 78(11):1173–6.
[34] Jones LM, Legge M, Goulding A. Factor analysis of the metabolic syndrome in spinal cord-injured men. Metab Clin Exp 2004;53(10):1372–7.
[35] Shetty KR, Sutton CH, Rudman IW, et al. Lipid and lipoprotein abnormalities in young quadriplegic men. Am J Med Sci 1992;303(4):213–6.
[36] Schmid A, Halle M, Stutzle C, et al. Lipoproteins and free plasma catecholamines in spinal cord injured men with different injury levels. Clin Physiol 2000;20(4):304–10.
[37] Summers SA, Garza LA, Zhou H, et al. Regulation of insulin-stimulated glucose transporter GLUT4 translocation and Akt kinase activity by ceramide. Mol Cell Biol 1998;18(9): 5457–64.
[38] Hotamisligil GS, Murray DL, Choy LN, et al. Tumor necrosis factor [alpha] inhibits signaling from the insulin receptor. Proc Natl Acad Sci U S A 1994;91(11):4854–8.
[39] Bauman WA, Spungen AM, Adkins RH, et al. Metabolic and endocrine changes in persons aging with spinal cord injury. Assist Technol 1999;11(2):88–96.
[40] Zhong YG, Levy E, Bauman WA. The relationships among serum uric-acid, plasma-insulin, and serum-lipoprotein levels in subjects with spinal-cord injury. Horm Metab Res 1995; 27(6):283–6.
[41] Huang Z, Willett WC, Manson JE, et al. Body weight, weight change, and risk for hypertension in women. Ann Intern Med 1998;128(2):81–8.
[42] Wofford MR, Hall JE. Pathophysiology and treatment of obesity hypertension. Curr Pharm Des 2004;10(29):3621–37.

[43] Engeli S, Negrel R, Sharma AM. Physiology and pathophysiology of the adipose tissue renin-angiotensin system. Hypertension 2000;35(6):1270–7.

[44] Castro JP, El-Atat FA, McFarlane SI, et al. Cardiometabolic syndrome: pathophysiology and treatment. Curr Hypertens Rep 2003;5(5):393–401.

[45] Weaver FM, Collins EG, Kurichi J, et al. Prevalence of obesity and high blood pressure in veterans with spinal cord injuries and disorders—a retrospective review. Am J Phys Med Rehabil 2007;86(1):22–9.

[46] Mavri A, Stegnar M, Krebs M, et al. Impact of adipose tissue on plasma plasminogen activator inhibitor-1 in dieting obese women. Arterioscler Thromb Vasc Biol 1999;19(6):1582–7.

[47] Aso Y, Wakabayashi S, Yamamoto R, et al. Metabolic syndrome accompanied by hypercholesterolemia is strongly associated with proinflammatory state and impairment of fibrinolysis in patients with type 2 diabetes: synergistic effects of plasminogen activator inhibitor-1 and thrombin-activatable fibrinolysis inhibitor. Diabetes Care 2005;28(9): 2211–6.

[48] Aubert H, Frere C, Aillaud MF, et al. Weak and non-independent association between plasma TAFI antigen levels and the insulin resistance syndrome. J Thromb Haemost 2003; 1(4):791–7.

[49] Alberti K, Zimmet PZ. Definition, diagnosis and classification of diabetes mellitus and its complications part 1: diagnosis and classification of diabetes mellitus—provisional report of a WHO consultation. Diabet Med 1998;15(7):539–53.

[50] Third Report of the National Cholesterol Education Program (NCEP) Expert panel on detection, evaluation, and treatment of high blood cholesterol in adults (Adult Treatment Panel III) Final Report. Circulation 2002;106(25):3143–421.

[51] International DF. Worldwide definition of the metabolic syndrome; 2005.

[52] Fitzgerald SG, Kellerher AM. Mobility challenges in individuals with a spinal cord injury with increased body weight. Top Spinal Cord Inj Rehabil 2007;12(4):54–63.

[53] Ballinger DA, Rintala DH, Hart KA. The relation of shoulder pain and range-of-motion problems to functional limitations, disability, and perceived health of men with spinal cord injury: a multifaceted longitudinal study. Arch Phys Med Rehabil 2000;81(12): 1575–81.

[54] Boninger ML, Cooper RA, Koontz AM, et al. Shoulder magnetic resonance imaging abnormalities, wheelchair propulsion, and gender. Arch Phys Med Rehabil 2003;84(11):1615–20.

[55] Cooper RA, Boninger ML, Shimada SD, et al. Glenohumeral joint kinematics and kinetics for three coordinate system representations during wheelchair propulsion. Am J Phys Med Rehabil 1999;78(5):435–46.

[56] Curtis KA, Drysdale GA, Lanza D, et al. Shoulder pain in wheelchair users with tetraplegia and paraplegia. Arch Phys Med Rehabil 1999;80(4):453–7.

[57] Dyson-Hudson TA, Kirshblum SC. Shoulder pain in chronic spinal cord injury, part I: epidemiology, etiology, and pathomechanics. J Spinal Cord Med 2004;27(1):4–17.

[58] Escobedo EM, Hunter JC, Hollister MC, et al. MR imaging of rotator cuff tears in individuals with paraplegia. AJR Am J Roentgenol 1997;168(4):919–23.

[59] Goldstein B, Young J, Escobedo EM. Rotator cuff repairs in individuals with paraplegia. Am J Phys Med Rehabil 1997;76(4):316–22.

[60] Lal S. Premature degenerative shoulder changes in spinal cord injury patients. Spinal Cord 1998;36(3):186–9.

[61] Samuelsson KAM, Tropp H, Gerdle B. Shoulder pain and its consequences in paraplegic spinal cord-injured, wheelchair users. Spinal Cord 2004;42(1):41–6.

[62] Sie IH, Waters RL, Adkins RH, et al. Upper extremity pain in the postrehabilitation spinal-cord injured patient. Arch Phys Med Rehabil 1992;73(1):44–8.

[63] Becker J, Nora DB, Gomes I, et al. An evaluation of gender, obesity, age and diabetes mellitus as risk factors for carpal tunnel syndrome. Clin Neurophysiol 2002;113(9):1429–34.

[64] Bland JDP. The relationship of obesity, age, and carpal tunnel syndrome: more complex than was thought? Muscle Nerve 2005;32(4):527–32.

[65] Karpitskaya Y, Novak CB, Mackinnon SE. Prevalence of smoking, obesity, diabetes mellitus, and thyroid disease in patients with carpal tunnel syndrome. Ann Plast Surg 2002;48(3): 269–73.
[66] Aljure J, Eltorai I, Bradley WE, et al. Carpal-tunnel syndrome in paraplegic patients. Paraplegia 1985;23(3):182–6.
[67] Gellman H, Sie I, Waters RL. Late complications of the weight-bearing upper extremity in the paraplegic patient. Clin Orthop Relat Res 1988;233:132–5.
[68] Boninger ML, Souza AL, Cooper RA, et al. Propulsion patterns and pushrim biomechanics in manual wheelchair propulsion. Arch Phys Med Rehabil 2002;83(5):718–23.
[69] Boninger ML, Impink BG, Cooper RA, et al. Relation between median and ulnar nerve function and wrist kinematics during wheelchair propulsion. Arch Phys Med Rehabil 2004;85(7):1141–5.
[70] Lohman TG. Advances in body composition assessment. Champaign (IL): Human kinetics; 1992.
[71] Gater D, Clasey J. Body composition assessment in spinal cord injury clinical trials. Top Spinal Cord Inj Rehabil 2006;11(3):36–49.
[72] Clasey JL, Gater DR. A comparison of hydrostatic weighing plethysmography in adults with spinal and air displacement cord injury. Arch Phys Med Rehabil 2005;86(11):2106–13.
[73] Bulbulian R, Johnson RE, Gruber JJ, et al. Body composition in paraplegic male athletes. Med Sci Sports Exerc 1987;19:195–201.
[74] Desport JC, Preux PM, Guinvarc'h S, et al. Total body water and percentage fat mass measurements using bioelectrical impedance analysis and anthropometry in spinal cord-injured patients. Clin Nutr 2000;19(3):185–90.
[75] George CM, Wells CL, Dugan NL, et al. Hydrostatic weights of patients with spinal cord injury. Phys Ther 1987;67:921–5.
[76] Jones LM, Legge M, Goulding A. Healthy body mass index values often underestimate body fat in men with spinal cord injury. Arch Phys Med Rehabil 2003;84(7):1068–71.
[77] Maggioni M, Bertoli S, Margonato V, et al. Body composition assessment in spinal cord injury subjects. Acta Diabetol 2003;40:S183–6.
[78] Modlesky CM, Bickel CS, Slade JM, et al. Assessment of skeletal muscle mass in men with spinal cord injury using dual-energy X-ray absorptiometry and magnetic resonance imaging. J Appl Physiol 2004;96(2):561–5.
[79] Monroe MB, Tataranni PA, Pratley R, et al. Lower daily energy expenditure as measured by a respiratory chamber in subjects with spinal cord injury compared with control subjects. Am J Clin Nutr 1998;68(6):1223–7.
[80] Chen Y, Henson S, Jackson AB, et al. Obesity intervention in persons with spinal cord injury. Spinal Cord 2006;44(2):82–91.
[81] Mollinger LA, Spurr GB, El Ghatit AZ. Daily energy expenditure and basal metabolic rates of patients with spinal cord injury. Arch Phys Med Rehabil 1999;66:420–6.
[82] Phillips E, Gater D. A practical approach for the nutritional management of obesity in spinal cord injury. Top Spinal Cord Inj Rehabil 2007;12(4):64–75.
[83] US Department of Agriculture. Center for nutrition policy and prevention. Dietary Guidelines for Americans; 2005.
[84] Saris WHM, Astrup A, Prentice AM, et al. Randomized controlled trial of changes in dietary carbohydrate/fat ratio and simple vs complex carbohydrates on body weight and blood lipids: the CARMEN study. Int J Obes 2000;24(10):1310–8.
[85] Wadden TA, Foster GD, Letizia KA. One-year behavioral treatment of obesity—comparison of moderate and severe caloric restriction and the effects of weight maintenance therapy. J Consult Clin Psychol 1994;62(1):165–71.
[86] McCrory MA, Fuss PJ, Hays NP, et al. Overeating in America: association between restaurant food consumption and body fatness in healthy adult men and women ages 19 to 80. Obes Res 1999;7(6):564–71.

[87] Gater D. Spinal cord injury. In: Ehrman JK, Gordon PM, Visich PS, et al, editors. Clinical exercise physiology. Champaign (IL): Human Kinetics; 2003. p. 503–26.
[88] Jacobs PL, Nash MS. Exercise recommendations for individuals with spinal cord injury. Sports Med 2004;34(11):727–51.
[89] Nash M, Gater D. Exercise to reduce obesity in SCI. Top Spinal Cord Inj Rehabil 2007; 12(4):76–93.
[90] Bauman WA, Alexander LR, Zhong YG, et al. Stimulated leg ergometry training improves body composition and HDL-cholesterol values. J Am Paraplegia Soc 1994;17(4):201.
[91] Hjeltnes N, Aksnes AK, Birkeland KI, et al. Improved body composition after 8 wk of electrically stimulated leg cycling in tetraplegic patients. Am J Physiol Regul Integr Comp Physiol 1997;42(3):R1072–9.
[92] Arterburn DE, Crane PK, Veenstra DL. The efficacy and safety of sibutramine for weight loss—a systematic review. Arch Intern Med 2004;164(9):994–1003.
[93] Li ZP, Maglione M, Tu WL, et al. Meta-analysis: pharmacologic treatment of obesity. Ann Intern Med 2005;142(7):532–46.
[94] Snow V, Barry P, Fitterman N, et al. Pharmacologic and surgical management of obesity in primary care: a clinical practice guideline from the American College of Physicians. Ann Intern Med 2005;142(7):525–31.
[95] Haddock CK, Poston WSC, Dill PL, et al. Pharmacotherapy for obesity: a quantitative analysis of four decades of published randomized clinical trials. Int J Obes 2002;26(2):262–73.

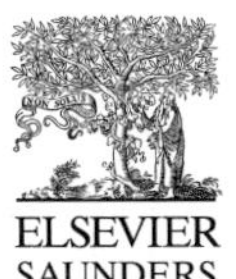

ELSEVIER
SAUNDERS

Phys Med Rehabil Clin N Am
18 (2007) 353–360

PHYSICAL MEDICINE
AND REHABILITATION
CLINICS OF
NORTH AMERICA

Index

Note: Page numbers of article titles are in **boldface** type.

1047-9651/07/$ - see front matter
doi:10.1016/S1047-9651(07)00043-5

N

O

R

S

T

U

V

W